- Are you of

- Do you find
  able to con

- Do you feel run-down, unhealthy, or
  "old before your time?"

- Does the idea of using caffeine or other
  stimulants concern you?

IF YOU ANSWERED "YES" TO ANY
OF THESE QUESTIONS,
LEARN THE SECRETS OF ONE OF
THE MOST POPULAR HERBAL
SUPPLEMENTS ON THE MARKET.

LEARN THE
SECRETS OF GINSENG

SECRETS
of
GINSENG

WINIFRED CONKLING

St. Martin's Paperbacks

SECRETS OF GINSENG

Copyright © 1999 by Cader Company, Inc.

All rights reserved. No part of this book may be used or reproduced in any manner whatsoever without written permission except in the case of brief quotations embodied in critical articles or reviews. For information address St. Martin's Press, 175 Fifth Avenue, New York, N.Y. 10010.

ISBN: 0-312-97072-2

Printed in the United States of America

St. Martin's Paperbacks edition / June 1999

10 9 8 7 6 5 4 3 2 1

For Louise Moore

Author's Note

This book is for informational purposes only. It is not intended to take the place of medical advice from a trained medical professional. Readers are advised to consult a physician or other qualified health professional regarding treatment of all of their health problems or before acting on any of the information or advice in this book. The fact that an organization or Web site is mentioned in this book as a source of information or herbs does not mean that the author or publisher recommends it.

Contents

Contents

Introduction

No single herb can be considered a panacea or a cure-all, but ginseng comes close. It is almost impossible to exaggerate the importance of ginseng's curative properties; for thousands of years, it has been used to enhance overall health and to treat various medical problems. Even ginseng's assigned botanical name, *Panax ginseng*, literally means "all healing."

Consider ginseng's impressive list of accomplishments. This treasured herb has been used for centuries to boost energy, sharpen the mind, reduce stress, reverse impotence, and extend life. It has also been used to enhance the immune system, control blood pressure, regulate blood-sugar levels, and strengthen the cardiovascular system. Because of its impressive track record in treating so many medical conditions, ginseng has been called "the root of life," "the divine herb," "the queen of the orient," "the prince of plants," "the longevity herb," "the wonder root," and "the king of herbs."

How can one herb do so much and earn so many accolades? The most likely explanation of ginseng's vast healing powers is that it is an adaptogen, or a "tonic" herb. Herbalists use these terms to describe herbs that help improve overall health and restore the body to balance during periods of physical or mental stress. Adaptogens also help boost resistance to disease; ginseng stimulates the immune system, which in turn strengthens the body in its fight against cancer, heart disease, diabetes, and other health problems. Even among adaptogens, ginseng stands out; it is considered the most respected and effective adaptogenic herb.

Because it is an adaptogen, ginseng alone is rarely used to "cure" any specific medical condition or health problem. Instead, it is a vital ingredient in literally thousands of healing herbal formulas or remedies. Ginseng's power as an adaptogen is what makes it such a revered herb in Oriental medicine, where it is credited with balancing or restoring *qi,* or vital life energy. Traditional Chinese Medicine classifies ginseng a "superior" medicine because its primary purpose is to balance, harmonize, and strengthen the body's various systems; in other words, ginseng helps the body heal itself.

This book will let you in on the secrets of ginseng and introduce you to the numerous health benefits attributed to the herb. **But before you embark on any self-care regimen you should first discuss it with your physician.** *Secrets of Ginseng* is divided into three main sections.

- Part 1, "Understanding Ginseng," outlines the history and folklore surrounding this world-famous herb. It also describes the various types of ginseng and explains how the active ingredients work to make the herb effective.

- Part 2, "The Healing Power of Ginseng," describes how the herb can be used to boost energy, reduce stress, enhance the immune system, and improve sexual function, among other uses.

- Part 3, "Using Ginseng," offers advice on buying and using the herb. It also provides advice on when and how to use ginseng to meet your particular health needs. The final chapter will help you design a program for using ginseng to address your particular health concerns and to improve your overall health.

The book also includes lists of organizations of interest, mail-order sources of herbs, and Web sites of interest. Those interested in additional reading will find books and articles of interest in the bibliography section.

The information in this book is based on both ancient wisdom and cutting-edge science. It includes knowledge that has been passed down for thousands of years by herbalists experienced in the use of ginseng as well the findings of research scientists who conduct their studies at leading medical facilities. In other words, this book explores the virtues and limitations of ginseng from both Eastern and Western perspectives. With this comprehensive approach, you will be able to appreciate the special qualities of this unique herb and choose how you would like to use ginseng to enhance your overall health and well-being.

PART ONE

Understanding Ginseng

CHAPTER 1

A Natural Wonder: The History, Folklore, and Legends of Ginseng

Herbalists have long considered ginseng one of the most useful and effective herbs. More than two thousand years ago, a group of Chinese herbalists prepared the first written classification of herbs, *The Pharmacopoeia of the Heavenly Husbandman*. (The "Divine Husbandman" is a legendary figure who is believed to have introduced agriculture, animal husbandry, and herbal medicine to the Chinese.) The book was a compilation of medical wisdom and remedies that had been passed down from as far back as 1800 B.C. Of the 252 herbs described, ginseng was rated the highest among the "superior" herbs, or the herbs that can be used on an ongoing basis to keep the body balanced and healthy.

At that time, ginseng's healing powers were well respected, and the herb was one of the main ingredients in hundreds of formulas in traditional Chinese medicine. A revision of the *Pharmacopoeia* by Tao Hung-Ching in the fifth century A.D. includes the following passage about ginseng's broad restorative powers: "It grows in the gorges of the mountains. It is used for repairing the five viscera, quieting the spirit, curbing the emotions, stopping agitation, removing noxious influences, brightening the eyes, enlightening the mind, and increasing wisdom. Continuous use leads on to longevity with light weight." As this early description indicates, ginseng was credited with healing the person as a whole rather than simply treating a single symptom or physical complaint.

The use of ginseng in holistic healing—the treatment of the body as an interconnected system—gained further credibility because of the shape of the root itself. The ancient Chinese often referred to ginseng as the "man root" because the shape of the branched root often resembles the human form. The Chinese believed that this indicated that the root could be used to treat the whole body. In fact, the word "ginseng" is derived from the words *jen shen*, meaning a crystallization of the essence of the earth (*shen*) in the form of a man (*jen*). Few modern herbalists would attribute ginseng's amazing healing powers to its shape, but the Chinese were right in that ginseng is a powerful herb that is effective in treating the body as a whole.

IN CELEBRATION OF GINSENG

Because of its treasured place as a healing herb, ginseng has been celebrated in mythology, folklore, and song in many cultures. Consider these examples of cultural reverence for "the king of herbs."

• Korean myth holds that ginseng was discovered by a young boy who spent his days taking care of his tired and ailing grandfather. One night the boy couldn't fall asleep, so he lit a candle in the room so that he could finish some chores. The candle repeatedly blew out, although he relit it several times. The boy determined that the candle was being extinguished without wind, so he concluded that a spirit must be present in the room. According to the story, the boy took a needle and thread and, when he felt the presence of the spirit in the room, he stabbed the needle in that direction. The needle disappeared, but when the boy followed the thread that had been attached to it, he found the needle stuck in the ground into a wild ginseng plant. The boy dug up the ginseng root and prepared a decoction for his grandfather, who then recovered from his illness and regained his vitality. According to the myth, the healing spirit of the ginseng plant rewarded the boy for his attentive and loving care of his grandfather.

- Finding wild ginseng was considered so difficult that people who hunted for the herb continually prayed to the spirits that were said to guard it. In Korea, ginseng hunters were said to keep "chaste and pure" for one week before an expedition and to pray that the ginseng spirits would look favorably on their hunt. During the actual hunt, senior members of the village would creep silently through the forest, using sign language and stepping carefully out of fear that they would offend or startle the spirits guarding the ginseng plants.

• When hunting for ginseng roots, the ancient Chinese would recite the following chant to the spirit of the jen-shen root:

> O great spirit! Do not go away
> I have come with a clean heart
> My soul is unstained
> It is purged of sin and wicked design
> Remain here, O greatest of spirits.

• Ancient Indian scriptures also mention the use of ginseng in healing. Indian hymns from five thousand years ago describe ginseng as "the root which is dug from the earth and which strengthens the nerves." In more poetic terms the ginseng hymn continues: "The strength of the horse, the mule, the goat, the ram, moreover the strength of the bull it bestows on him. This herb will make thee so full of lusty strength that thou shalt, when excited, exhale heat as a thing on fire."

GINSENG'S INFLUENCE SPREADS

The modern story of ginseng began in the early eighteenth century when Father Jartoux, a Jesuit missionary working in China, became interested in the plant. Father Jartoux became curious about the herb when he met some ginseng collectors of the Chinese emperor Kanghi near the Chinese-Korean border. The collectors gave him four samples of the medicinal roots. When the priest tried them, he felt energized; his pulse raced and he felt vigorous and strong. During another outing, Father Jartoux allegedly went horseback riding with the Chinese emperor. The priest rode nearly to exhaustion; then, supposedly, the emperor gave him half a ginseng root to chew. After biting into the root, the priest felt reinvigo-

HERBAL INSURANCE

Mature, wild ginseng roots can be worth thousands of dollars a piece. Rather than investing in mutual funds or individual retirement accounts, some Chinese people buy these roots as an insurance policy for their old age. Unlike a conventional investment, a high-quality ginseng root offers the dual advantages of being an asset that can be sold to raise money if needed in old age—or consumed if the individual needs to partake of the herb's healing powers. If it is stored in an airtight container, a ginseng root can retain its potency indefinitely.

rated and continued with the ride.

Impressed with ginseng's potency, in 1714 Father Jartoux published a paper titled "The Description of the Tartarian Plant Ginseng" in the *Philosophical Transactions of the Royal Society of London*. In the paper he reported that after taking ginseng, "I found my pulse much fuller and quicker . . . I found myself much more vigorous and could bear labour much better and easier than before." He also wrote that "if ginseng is to be found in any other country in the world, it may be particularly in Canada, where the forest and mountains very much resemble these here [in China]."

Another Jesuit priest, Father Joseph Francis Lafitau, read the article on ginseng in Montreal, Canada, where he worked as a missionary with Mohawk Indians. He asked the Native Americans if they were familiar with the herb; they showed him a similar plant, American ginseng (*Panax quinquefolium*). At that time, a number of North American Indian tribes used ginseng in rituals involving healing and spirit guidance.

Father Lafitau sent root samples to Father Jartoux, who shared them with Chinese herbalists. The Chinese took great interest in the American ginseng and were eager to buy more. The French hired the Native Americans to collect the herb for export to China. Word of the profitable overseas market spread from Canada to the colonies, and within several years ginseng became an established and lucrative export. Oriental herbalists valued American ginseng for its different energetic properties compared to Asian ginseng.

Once North American fur traders and trappers learned that ginseng—often referred to as "shang"—was a valuable export, they began collecting it from the wilderness. It is said that Daniel Boone made more money from selling ginseng than from selling animal hides. Ginseng soon became an important part of the American economy; many settlers supported themselves and their families by digging ginseng roots. China offered an unlimited market for ginseng, and the profits were so great that ginseng was second only to the fur trade in profitability. In 1862 more than 620,000 pounds of dried ginseng roots were shipped to Asia from the United States.

GINSENG IN AMERICA

In addition to being a popular export, ginseng was a common herbal medicine in America, especially in the nineteenth cen-

GINSENG AND NATIVE AMERICANS

Many Native Americans appreciated the therapeutic powers of ginseng. While it is difficult to distinguish which uses of the herb originated with the Native Americans and which were learned from the settlers, the following list provides a reasonable idea of ways different Native American tribes used ginseng:

- Crow: to facilitate childbirth

- Cherokee: to relieve headaches, muscle cramps, and menstrual cramps

- Creek: to stop bleeding, relieve sore throats, reduce fever

- Houmas: to stop vomiting

- Iroquois: to promote overall health, to revive a person after fainting

- Meskwakis: to improve overall health and mental powers

- Mohawks: to reduce fever

- Penobscot: to increase female fertility

- Pottawatomis: to relieve earache and sore eyes

- Sac-Fox: to improve overall health

- Seminole: to ease breathing

- Seneca: to strengthen the overall health of the elderly

tury. Ginseng was listed in the official book of medicine, the *U.S. Pharmacopoeia*, from 1842 to 1882 as a stimulant and a digestive aid.

American interest in ginseng decreased in the late nineteenth century, when consumers became skeptical of herbal tonics in general. During this time, there was a lot of consumer health fraud, and ginseng's reputation was tainted by the misrepresentation of many commercial products. Understandably, ginseng fell out of favor with most Americans, who were not able to distinguish ginseng's authentic healing powers from the exaggerated and outright false claims made by many producers of herbal tonics.

While American consumption of ginseng diminished, the export business did not.

But after decades of overharvesting, wild ginseng had become scarce. By the end of the nineteenth century, farmers began to cultivate ginseng as a crop. However, ginseng can be difficult to grow because it is easily damaged by worms, pests, and fungi. (Today most American ginseng is grown in Wisconsin, Michigan, and the Appalachian Mountains, where the winters are cold enough for the plant to enter a period of dormancy.)

While ginseng production and export continued, most American researchers and healers lost interest in ginseng. A few studies were done on the healing power of the herb in the early twentieth century, but for the most part there was little scientific interest in ginseng until 1949, when a researcher named Dr. Itskovity I. Brekhman began conducting studies at the Institute of Biologically Active Substances at the Soviet Union's Academy of Sciences in Vladivostok, Russia. Brekhman was especially interested in ginseng medicinal qualities. He conducted hundreds of studies on ginseng and other adaptogens. In explaining his special interest in ginseng, he noted: "Ginseng has been used as a remedy for 5,000 years. During those fifty centuries, numerous generations, social systems, medical doctrines, and medicines have sunk into oblivion, yet, ginseng still exists. It exists despite the fact that science not only ignored, but rejected it." Over the next sixteen years, Brekhman focused his attention on ginseng and did a lot of impressive research. His work marks the beginning of modern medicine's serious exploration of ginseng's healing powers. His research also encouraged other scientists to explore the herb. Today Brekhman's tests have been replicated at a number of universities, including the University of Minnesota, the University of Illinois, and the University of California at Los Angeles.

To date, more than three thousand scientific studies have been conducted on ginseng and its active ingredients. While many of these studies have documented the myriad health benefits attributed to the herb, even modern scientists do not fully understand how ginseng works.

A WORD ABOUT HERBS

Ginseng is one of Mother Nature's most effective herbal remedies or botanicals. Herbs are often safer, cheaper, and more effective than synthetic drugs, and they can be used to treat a handful of conditions that mainstream medicines can't touch. That's not to say that man-made drugs have no place in your medicine cabinet; they do. But in many cases herbal remedies such as ginseng can complement conventional medicine and add another dimension to your health care.

Despite the fact that herbs are natural, they can be strong medicine. Many people who agonize over taking an over-the-counter pain-killer think nothing of swallowing an herbal treatment because they consider it "natural" and therefore not dangerous. But herbs that have the ability to heal also have the ability to harm, if misused. While in general herbal remedies are safer and have fewer side effects than man-made drugs, they can be as potent and harmful as synthetic drugs, and they should be treated with the same respect.

Part of the confusion about safety stems from the way herbal treatments are labeled. Unlike synthetic drugs, herbal remedies do not have to go through the formal approval process of the U.S. Food and Drug Administration because they are classified as foods or food additives rather than drugs. This means that manufacturers of herbal remedies must be cautious about the claims they make on their package labels—drug-related claims and warning are prohibited. Consumers must be on their toes about understanding the products they are buying. It's up to you to read the package directions.

You can find ginseng and other herbal remedies in health food stores, but recently they have been showing up in conventional supermarkets and pharmacies as well. If you can't find what you need at local stores, or you want to buy whole, unprocessed ginseng roots, see the information on mail-order companies on pages 229–233.

CHAPTER 2

Getting to Know Ginseng: Recognizing Types of Ginseng

While the term "ginseng" often is used to describe a number of different herbs, botanically and medicinally speaking, the only true ginsengs are the plants in the *Panax* genus within the Araliaceae family. (The Araliaceae family also includes sarsparilla, ivy, and Indian roots, among others.)

There are several different species of ginseng, many with different medicinal qualities. The most common types are:

- Asian ginseng *(Panax ginseng)*: The term "ginseng" is used most often to describe Asian ginseng, which is also called Oriental, Chinese, or Korean ginseng. These names are designed to draw the distinction between Asian and American ginseng, which have different qualities and affect the body in different ways.

Asian ginseng is the herb used most often in medical tests on the efficacy of ginseng.

- American ginseng *(Panax quinquefolius)*: This herb grows wild in North America, from as far north as Quebec to as far south as Florida. The herb was used by Native Americans to treat indigestion, sore eyes, earache, menstrual cramps, fever, and bronchitis. Today most American ginseng is cultivated in Wisconsin, Michigan, the Appalachian mountains and Canada and shipped to the Orient after harvest. Ninety-five percent of the American-grown ginseng is sold overseas, primarily to Hong Kong, China, Korea, and Japan. The U.S. exports over 2 million pounds of ginseng a year.

- Dwarf ginseng *(Panax trifolius)*: This rare type of American ginseng grows mostly in the southern Appalachian Mountains. Native Americans used the roots of this herb to treat headaches and nervous conditions; they used the whole plant to treat cough, indigestion, gout, hepatitis, hives, rheumatism, and skin problems. It is sometimes called ground-nut because of the root's round shape. (This form of ginseng doesn't have the traditional "man-shaped" root.)

- Korean ginseng: Korean ginseng is the same as Asian ginseng. The name change is an attempt to develop business for Korean ginseng growers so that they could compete better with Chinese growers. Korean ginseng can be thought of as a "brand name" rather than a separate species of plant.

- Sanchi ginseng (*Panax notoginseng*, also called *Panax pseudoginseng*, variety *notoginseng*): Unlike Asian ginseng with five leaves, this type of ginseng has seven leaves. (The word Sanchi means "seven.") This plant is sometimes called pseudoginseng because its roots and flowers can be used in place of Panax ginseng as a tonic, although it is not considered an adaptogen. Unlike Asian and American ginseng, pseudoginseng is not as effective as an overall tonic. Instead, this herb often is used in Chinese hospitals to stop bleeding, disperse blood in bruises, reduce pain, and decrease swelling when treating emergencies.

- Himalayan ginseng *(Panax pseudoginseng* subsp. *Himalaicus)*: This subspecies of ginseng grows in Tibet and is rarely available in North America. The plant's ginsenoside content—the amount of active medicine it contains— falls in between that of Chinese and Japanese ginseng. Himalayan healers often use this plant to help people with poor appetites and digestive problems.

- Japanese ginseng *(Panax japonicus)*: Japanese herbalists often use it in place of Asian ginseng in their formulas. Above the ground, Asian and Japanese ginsengs are virtually identical, but their roots grow quite differently. Japanese ginseng roots grow as a mass of roots extending from a central rhizome rather than being shaped like a man. Researchers have found that Japanese ginseng contains similar ingredients to Asian ginseng but in different proportions. Chinese herbalists consider Japanese ginseng less powerful, but they recommend it for people they consider too ill to tolerate the powerful stimulation associated with Asian ginseng.

- Siberian ginseng *(Eleutherococcus senticosus)*: Siberian ginseng belongs to the Araliaceae family but is not a true ginseng of the *Panax* genus. It is a much larger bush with prickly stems that grows in Siberia, as the name implies. Siberian ginseng shares many of the healing properties of the true ginsengs, but because it is not a true ginseng, many herbalists refer to it by its formal name, Eleutherococcus, or somewhat more casually as "Eleuthero." Siberian ginseng often is sold as a cheaper alternative to the more expensive Panax ginsengs. Eleutherococcus works in the body like a mild form of Asian ginseng. Chinese researchers who have compared it to Asian ginseng find that it is a mildly stimulating tonic that is effective in balancing metabolic energy, but overall it is much less effective at increasing vitality and general feelings of well-being. Siberian ginseng contains compounds known as eueutherosides. While not the same as the ginsenosides found in Asian and American ginseng, they share some chemical properties.

THE PLANTS

Even among the true ginsengs, the plants themselves have different physical characteristics. Following are descriptions of the major ginseng plants:

- Asian ginseng has five saw-toothed leaves on the top of a straight stalk. The plant can grow eight to thirty inches tall; older plants can have two or three separate stalks. When the plant is about three or four years old, it forms pale green-white flowers, which produce red berries. The roots can grow to one and one-half inches in diameter and four inches in length.

- American ginseng is a somewhat smaller plant with seven leaves that are narrower than the leaves on the Asian plant. It is found in shaded forests of the Northeast, especially under beech and maple trees. The plant has been cultivated successfully in China, where it is quite popular. This plant has three large leaves and two small leaves from the same stem. It generates yellowish-green flowers and red berries. Its roots tend to be up to one inch thick and three inches long.

- Siberian ginseng grows in elevations up to 2,500 feet and in forests at lower elevations. It has thorn-covered stems and flowers of yellow or violet, followed by black berries.

The medicinal part of all ginseng plants is the thick, fleshy root, which looks something like a white or yellow carrot. The root tends to be branched or curled and often numerous tendrils or rootlets grow from the main root. The top of the root has a crinkled neck, which contains the buds for the next year's growth. Ginseng is a deciduous perennial; the leaves and stalks die each fall, and the new stems sprout from the root in April or May. Each time the plant passes through this cycle of growth and decay, a new wrinkle forms on the neck of the root, making assessing the age of the plant easy.

Wild ginseng used to grow in the forests of China, Korea, and the former Soviet Union, but due to its popularity, wild roots are now exceedingly rare. The herb has been domesticated, and it is cultivated throughout eastern Asia. The most significant problem with cultivated ginseng is that pesticides often are sprayed on commercial plants.

YIN AND YANG: AMERICAN AND ASIAN GINSENG

While Asian and American ginseng may share a branch on the family tree, they have very different effects on the human body. In traditional Chinese medicine, the different types of ginseng are believed to possess different characteristics, and they are used for different healing purposes.

Using the terminology of Oriental medicine, Asian ginseng is "yang," while American ginseng is "yin." These differences become clear when comparing the characteristics of both plants.

- Asian ginseng is considered a warm, stimulating "yang" tonic; it is best avoided by people who tend to be nervous or anxious, unless they are feeling exhausted or taking the tonic to offset conditions associated with aging. Asian ginseng is considered masculine, meaning it may accentuate male hormonal qualities. It tends to be more effective in males than females.

- American ginseng is a cooling, sedating "yin" tonic; it helps to bring balance and harmony to the body, reducing stress and encouraging calm. American ginseng is well suited for people who are active and

energetic—or anxious and nervous—
and want to use ginseng to slow down
rather than to rev their engines. Because
American ginseng has cooling properties, it often is used in place of Asian ginseng in hot climates and during the hot
summer months; likewise many people
prefer Asians ginseng in the cold winter
months because of its warming properties.

American ginseng is much more popular
in Asia than it is in the United States. Why
don't Americans appreciate the special
properties of home-grown ginseng? In part,
the answer involves the go-go American
culture that puts a premium on action, energy, and vitality. Americans tend to want
more zest for life, rather than calm and inner peace. On the other hand, people in
China and in Asia often use ginseng to
achieve inner balance and maintain vitality
in old age.

When it comes to using ginseng, you must
consider the condition you are treating
when selecting the appropriate plant. A

THE NOT-QUITE GINSENGS

Several other herbs are sometimes inaccurately referred to as ginseng. In some cases, these plants are called ginseng in attempt to confuse consumers; other times they are called ginseng because they do have some mild adaptogenic properties. The roll call of ginseng wannabes includes the following:

- Brazilian ginseng or suma (*Pfaffia paniculata*)
- California ginseng (*Aralia Californica*)
- False ginseng, dang shen, or "poor man's ginseng" (*Codonopsis pilosula*)
- Indian ginseng or ashwaganda (*Withiania somnifera*)
- Oregon ginseng or devil's club (*Opopanax horridum*)
- Prince's ginseng (*Pseudostellaria heterophylla*)
- Women's ginseng or dong quai (*Angelica sinensis or S. acutiloba*)

If a product labeled ginseng lists one or more of these herbs in its list of ingredients, choose another product. These herbs are not as effective as true ginseng.

young, active, fit person living in a warm climate probably would prefer to use the yin (sedating) American ginseng; an older person who tires easily and wants more energy for the day likely would opt for the yang (energizing) Asian ginseng. (For more information on choosing the right type of ginseng for your health concerns, see Chapter 10.)

THE TRUTH ABOUT AMERICAN "RED" GINSENG

Some American ginseng roots grown in Michigan and Wisconsin are steam-cured to turn them red in the same way that Asian ginseng roots are cured in China and Korea to alter their color. Some marketers try to claim these red roots are more valuable, but this is not true. Real wild American ginseng roots are never cured in this way because they are much more valuable in their natural state.

While the precise effects of curing on American ginseng is unknown, it is believed that steam-curing increases the warming properties of Chinese ginseng. The value of this practice with American roots is questionable because American ginseng's therapeutic value comes from its cooling and moistening properties. Steaming presumably would reduce these properties.

Another kind of "red ginseng" does not have the same medicinal value as the above herbs. Some companies in the Southwest market a plant commonly known as caniagre (*Rumex hymenosepalus*) as American red desert ginseng, Wild American red ginseng, or Hymenosephalus ginseng. Caniagre has a natural reddish-brown color resembling that of cured ginseng. But appearances can be deceptive. The herb has entirely different botanical and medicinal properties than ginseng, and it is useless as an adaptogen.

OTHER TONIC HERBS

While ginseng is the best-known and most effective tonic herb, others also have been found to have some adaptogenic properties. Many times these herbs are used in formulas that also contain ginseng.

Asparagus root (*Asparagus cochinchinensis*)
Astragalus (*Astragalus membranaceus*)
Atractylodes (*Atractylodes maacrocephala*)
Codonopsis (*Codonopsis pilosula*)

Cordyceps (*Cordyceps sinensis*)
Deer antler (*Cornu Cervi parvum*)
Dendrobium (*Dendrobium nobile*)
Dioscorea (*Dioscorea opposita*)
Dong quai (*Angelica sinensis*)
Eucommia (*Eucommia ulmoides*)
Fo-ti (*Polygonum multiflorum*)
Ganoderma (*Ganoderma lucidum*)
Glehnia (*Glehnia littoralis*)
Jujube dates, red dates (*Zizyphus jujuba*)
Licorice root (*Glycyrrhiza glabra*)
Ligustrum, privet (*Ligustrum lucidum*)
Lycium berries (*Lycium chinensis*)
Morindae (*Morinda officinalis*)
Peony (*Paeonia lactiflora*)
Poria (*Poria cocos*)
Prince ginseng (*Pseudostellaria heterophylla*)
Rehmannia (*Rehmannia glutinosa*)
Schizandra berries (*Schizandr sinensis*)
Tienchi ginseng, sanchi ginseng (*Panax pseudoginseng*)

Chapter 3

How Ginseng Works:
The Active Ingredients

For thousands of years, herbalists have appreciated and enjoyed the healing benefits of ginseng without fully understanding the biochemical intricacies of how the herb affects the body. Today we have a basic understanding of how ginseng works, but many of the subtle healing properties and relationships between various ingredients still remain a mystery. We don't know why ginseng works, but we know that it does.

For decades in the 20th century ginseng drew little attention from mainstream scientists. Superficial tests on the herb showed that it contained the expected range of ingredients: carbohydrates, cellulose, minerals, and other common plant materials. Few researchers thought much about ginseng until the early 1960s, when western scientists took note of a study done in the former

Soviet Union that showed that ginseng could increase the endurance and energy of mice in a laboratory setting. Intrigued about the prospect of isolating the active ingredients responsible for increasing stamina, a number of researchers began serious research on the herb. Specifically, they began to analyze and try to isolate the active ingredients in ginseng.

What they discovered were compounds known as terpenoidal glycosides. Specifically, these are sugar molecules (glycosides) attached to plant hormones (terpenoid molecules). Ginseng glycosides form in the leaves, flowers, and outer coating of the root, then they are stored in the root's fleshy part. As much as 2 to 6 percent of the dry root may consist of glycosides.

A Japanese researcher coined the term "ginsenoside" to describe these glycosides in 1961. (For a time, some researchers referred to them as "panaxosides," but ginsenoside is the accepted term today.) Glycosides occur in other types of plants, but ginsenosides occur only in the *Panax ginsengs*.

More than twenty different ginsenosides have been identified. They have been named Ra, Rb, Rc, and so on to distinguish one from another. The different types of ginsenosides vary in proportion, depending on the type of plant, where it is grown, how old it is, how it is dried and processed, among other variables. The older the root, the greater the concentration of ginsenosides, which accounts for the greater healing power—as well as the higher cost—of mature ginseng roots. Some ginsenosides take five or six years to develop, and some even longer. According to scientific analysis, the optimum time to harvest ginseng is when the roots are five to six years old.

In the laboratory, researchers have many of ginseng's healing in isolated ginsenosides, with different ginsenosides yielding different properties. For example, Re and Rb ginsenosides tend to be soothing and calming, while Re and Rg tend to be energizing and stimulating. The differences in the amounts and types of ginsenosides in various subspecies of ginseng help to explain the range of characteristics among the plants. For example, it explains how one ginseng plant (American ginseng) can be calming and quieting, while another (Asian ginseng) can be stimulating and arousing. (For more information on the the various characteristics of different ginseng plants, see Chapter 10.)

In addition to stimulating or soothing the central nervous system, ginsenosides have been found to cause other physical reactions. They have been shown to enhance muscle tone, regulate blood-sugar levels, affect the adrenal glands and hormones, and increase metabolism. The specific actions of the ginsenosides may be the key to the many healing properties associated with ginseng.

MORE IS NOT ALWAYS BETTER

From the ginseng user's point of view, isolating the ginsenosides offers a new opportunity for product comparison. In theory, a consumer can compare the relative amount of ginsenosides in various commercial products to determine which product is more potent. To build consumer confidence, some manufacturers have set standards for the amount of ginsenosides in their products. In fact, in 1987 the *Swiss Pharmacopoeia* set a standard that a product must contain at least 1 to 2 percent ginsenosides to be called pure ginseng.

Unfortunately, assessing the quality of ginseng isn't simply a matter of measuring the ginsenosides, and more is not always better. Some superior-quality roots have fewer ginsenosides than poor-quality roots. In addition, some roots with high levels of ginsenosides are of poor quality. For example, root hairs and tendrils are of poor quality and have less medicinal value, yet they contain very high levels of ginsenosides; and infected and damaged roots have higher levels of ginsenosides than healthy roots. Ginsenosides clearly play a role in the healing power of ginseng, but we do not fully understand exactly how these chemicals affect the medicinal value of the root.

At present, however, the ginsenoside level remains the best way we have to assess the quality of commercially prepared products. When comparing ginseng products, look for one with a high ginsenoside level, but again be aware that this does not ensure the roots are of optimal medicinal value. The only way to be sure the ginsenoside content comes from healthy, mature roots is to purchase whole roots. For more information on buying ginseng, see Chapter 9.

The overall effectiveness of ginseng is undoubtedly influenced by the other ingredients found in the plant. In addition to the ginsenosides, scientists have identified phenols (such as maltol), polysaccharides (sugar compounds that boost immunity), a protein material that assists in the metabolism of sugar and fat, vitamins (including A, B, and E), minerals (including calcium, magnesium, and phosphorus), alkaloids, mucilaginous compound, and other substances that may offer some healing benefits. While it is possible to isolate a number of these individual ingredients, it is likely that ginseng's effectiveness depends on the synergistic effect of all these components working together. When it comes to ginseng, as well as most other herbs, the whole is more effective than the sum of its parts.

ALL THAT AND VITAMINS, TOO

In addition to the active ingredients that give ginseng its healing powers, the herb is also an excellent source of several vitamins. Ginseng contains vitamin A (which helps support the mucous membranes, eyes and skin, and the all-important immune system), vitamin E (which is essential for a healthy heart and circulatory system), and the B-complex vitamins thiamin, riboflavin, B12, and niacin (which are critical for maintaining healthy nerves, skin, hair, eyes, liver, and gastrointestinal system). In addition, ginseng contains calcium, iron, phosphorus, sodium, silicon, potassium, manganese, and sulfur.

PART TWO

The Healing Power of Ginseng

CHAPTER 4

Ginseng and Energy

Ginseng is a safe, effective, and natural stimulant that can boost your energy without the agitation, jittery feelings, and other unpleasant side effects associated with other stimulants, such as caffeine, over-the-counter pick-me-up products, or prescription amphetamines. Ginseng can revitalize you both physically and mentally when you're feeling tired and run down. It also can provide an energy boost when you're facing the physical and mental challenges associated with hard physical work, studying for exams, or driving long distances.

Ginseng works as both a short-term stimulant and a long-term restorative. In addition to helping you overcome brief periods of fatigue or exhaustion, ginseng also is an effective tonic when it is taken consistently for months or years. According to traditional Chinese medicine, long-term ginseng use is especially helpful during recovery from disease as well as in countering fatigue associated with aging.

When ginseng is taken on an ongoing basis at a maintenance level, it not only helps to boost energy levels but also can ward off illness caused by weakened resistance. While it can be difficult to attribute signs of good health to a single herb, Chinese healers often credit ginseng with saving the lives of many seriously ill people and with helping people fight off life-threatening diseases.

Ginseng's potential as an energizing agent has drawn the attention of some governmental bodies, and it has been extensively studied by a number of countries. The Commission E, the German research body created to evaluate the safety and efficacy of herbal remedies, has decided that ginseng is a "tonic for invigoration and fortification in times of fatigue and debility, for declining capacity for work and concentration, and also during convalescence."

Ginseng has even made its mark on the space mission. During the early days of space travel, Soviet cosmonauts used ginseng as a stimulant. Soviet researchers had found that ginseng increased alertness and improved performance more successfully than synthetic drugs, and it did so without interfering with sleep or producing unpleasant side effects.

Ginseng also has been used by Soviet coaches and trainers to improve the performance of athletes in training. Studies conducted at the Legraft Institute of Physical Culture and Sports in the Soviet Union concluded that ginseng and related plants help the body recover after intense exercise and increase the body's resistance to disease. In fact, the sports ministry advised Soviet athletes to take ginseng to help overcome exhaustion and stress during training.

Indeed, ginseng has an impressive track record as both a stimulant and a tonic herb. While many Americans value ginseng most as a short-term pick-me-up and many Asians value it most as a long-term tonic or restorative herb, the truth is that ginseng is effective in both applications, as a number of studies show.

CONSIDER THE EVIDENCE

Some of the earliest experiments on ginseng's effectiveness as a stimulant were remarkably simple: Researchers put mice in extremely cold water and had them swim to the point of exhaustion. Researchers gave ginseng to half the mice; they found that the mice that were given ginseng were able to swim for nearly twice as long as the mice that were not given the herb. This study has been repeated time and again, always with the same results. The energizing effect of ginseng has been shown to occur even when the mice received moderate doses of ginseng, the equivalent of amounts a human might take for overall health maintenance.

The next question the researchers pondered was how long these energizing effects would last. They continued their research and found that the effect of the ginseng is cumulative. If the mice were given ginseng for one month, then the energizing effect of the herb lasted for two or three weeks after the animal stopped receiving the herb.

While these rodent swim meets might seem cruel or sadistic to an outsider, they offer objective evidence of the stimulating effects of ginseng. In human trials, researchers often were left to wonder whether the people involved in the study performed better because they expected to, the so-called placebo effect. The animal studies showed that the mice did not perform better due to any psychological influence or placebo factor but rather due to physiological changes in their bodies. Caffeine, antidepressant drugs, and other herbs also have been shown to be stimulants, but many of these agents have unwanted side effects not found with ginseng.

Experiments involving humans offer more directly relevant information, but it is important to control for the possibility that subjects could knowingly or unknowingly alter their behavior. These human studies affirmed the impressive findings of the animal research:

- One study involved proofreaders who were given ginseng then asked to concentrate on their work for longer periods of time than usual. Tests of speed and accuracy found that the ginseng-using proofreaders increased their workload by 12 percent while at the same time they made 5 percent fewer mistakes than the proofreaders given a dummy extract or placebo.

- A similar study involving Russian telegraph operators yielded equally impressive results. In two tests, the operators were asked to encode a special message quickly. The participants who were given a placebo increased their speed slightly in the second test, but they made 28 percent more errors. Those who took ginseng were faster and made 10 percent fewer mistakes.

- In a controlled study involving males between the ages of twenty and twenty-

four, the group that took ginseng extract
for twelve weeks had greater levels of attention, arithmetic mental processing,
and coordination and faster auditory reaction times than people in the control
group.

- In a German study of sixty people between the ages of twenty and seventy,
half were given a ginseng extract and half
were given a placebo. Both groups were
tested for visual acuity by using a flickering light test. Participants were asked
to point out when a flickering light is
flashing so fast that it appears to be continuously on. The group taking ginseng
had superior visual acuity (they could
see the flickers longer) compared to the
people in the control group.

- Another important study on ginseng's
ability to boost energy involved nurses in
London who were tested as they
switched from a day shift to a night shift.
The nurses who participated in the study
were given either Korean ginseng or a
dummy pill during the first three days of

the switch. After the third night, which tends to be the night they experience the most fatigue, the nurses were tested for performance, energy, tiredness, and ability to sleep during the day. Typically, the nurses experienced a decline in energy, alertness, and job performance after switching to the night shift. When given one gram of Korean ginseng for just three days, the nurses felt better and performed better than without it; they didn't reach the level of work on the day shift, but they made about a 50 percent improvement. The nurses didn't sleep well during the day (perhaps because the ginseng was stimulating), but they did tend to cope much better at night.

- Traditional Chinese medicine has considered ginseng a highly effective tonic for older people for thousands of years. This ancient wisdom has been affirmed by researchers from the University of Goteberg, Sweden, where 480 older volunteers were given either a ginseng-vitamin mixture or a dummy pill. The people taking ginseng were found to be more alert and more relaxed; they also scored higher than their peers who did not take ginseng in mood, energy, general well-being, and measures of overall quality of life. A similar study done in Mexico confirmed these results.

Interestingly, human studies have found that the effects of the ginseng vary depending on the physical condition of the person taking the herb. In general, the more tired a person feels, the more energizing the ginseng will be. When ginseng has been tested with young fit people, the results are less impressive than when it was tested with older people in greater need of a stimulant. In fact, ginseng offered no discernible benefits to the stamina and performance of young marathon runners, while it offered significant benefits to older, less-fit athletes. This finding makes sense; as a tonic herb, ginseng helps bring the body into balance, it does not endow the body with Herculean endurance or ability.

GINSENG AND THE CENTRAL NERVOUS SYSTEM

Ginseng revs up the nervous system and speeds reaction times and reflexes. Studies on both animals and humans have shown that ginseng actually increases the efficiency of cerebral activity, effectively helping the brain work faster and more accurately. A number of studies have shown impressive results of ginseng's ability to stimulate—but not to overstimulate—the brain and nervous system.

- Hundreds of animal studies (most involving mice and rats) have shown that ginseng improves learning ability. In one study, rats were given either ginseng or caffeine. The rats given ginseng learned faster than the caffeine-taking rats, and they tired less rapidly.

- Ginseng seems to improve recall of learned information. As part of several research projects, mice were allowed to learn a repetitive behavior pattern, then they were given time to forget it. After enough time had passed that the mice would not be expected to recall the lesson, they were given a single low dose of ginseng (the equivalent of less than a single gram in a human); these ginseng-taking mice remembered the information without further instruction, while the mice that did not receive the herb did not recall the information. The researchers concluded that ginseng stimulates the "basic neural processes," improving recall without causing any loss of equilibrium or excitability common with other stimulants.

• These brain-enhancing benefits associated with ginseng appear to be long lasting. Researchers have found that taking ginseng for 15 to 45 days increased mental functioning as well as physical endurance, both during the time the herb was taken and also for six weeks after participants stopped taking ginseng.

GINSENG AND PHYSICAL PERFORMANCE

Exercise is a critical part of good health, and ginseng actually can improve sports performance. Ginseng has been used to improve physical performance for more than two thousand years. Now modern research has confirmed that this energizing herb can actually help to increase physical stamina and exercise endurance. Consider the following information.

- According to Chinese folklore, the ancient Chinese had such confidence in ginseng's ability to improve athletic performance that it is said that they used physical tests to evaluate quality. Supposedly the Chinese determined the quality of ginseng by having two men— one with a ginseng root in his mouth and the other without—run about two miles. If the runner chewing the ginseng did not feel fatigued at the end of the race, the root was considered authentic. A contemporary version of this test was carried out in 1948 by Soviet researchers who took one hundred Soviet soldiers on a cross-country run in eastern Siberia. Half the soldiers received a ginseng extract a few hours before the run; the other received a placebo. Those who took the ginseng ran an average of 53 seconds faster than those not receiving the herb.

• Ginseng allows the body to work harder and more efficiently. An eight-week study conducted in Sweden on thirty-eight healthy men between the ages of fifty and fifty-four found that those who took ginseng had a significantly greater workload capacity than those who did not receive the herb. As part of the study, the men pedaled a stationary bicycle with an increasing workload until they reached the point of exhaustion. In addition to working harder, the men who received the ginseng also had lower heart rates.

- In a series of experiments involving Soviet Olympic athletes, thirty males and females took ginseng before sleep and again one hour before they began their morning workouts. The athletes—sprinters, high jumpers, runners, decathaletes, and marathoners—experienced higher levels of endurance, and they felt eager to train longer and harder, compared with the athletes in the group who did not receive ginseng. In addition, the pulse and blood pressure in the ginseng-taking athletes returned to normal faster after exercise than the measures did in the group that went herb-free.

- Ginseng allows the lungs to fill with air more completely. As part of one study, oxygen intake while resting increased almost 30 percent after one month of taking ginseng on a daily basis. In another experiment, a group of fourteen German athletes who took ginseng twice daily had significantly higher rates of oxygen utilization during the ten-week study, compared with the athletes who did not take ginseng.

SECRETS OF GINSENG

- In an experiment with Soviet runners, thirty-four participants were given 2 milligrams (mg) ginseng thirty minutes before a race, thirty-three were given 4 mg, and forty-one were given no ginseng. The results of the ten-kilometer race corresponded with the amount of ginseng given. The high-dose ginseng group finished in an average of forty-five minutes, the low-dose ginseng group in forty-nine minutes, and the no-ginseng group in fifty-three minutes.

- In a study in Switzerland, thirty highly trained athletes between the ages of eighteen and thirty-one were given ginseng, ginseng with vitamin E, or a placebo for nine weeks. Those who received the ginseng or the ginseng with vitamin E had substantially higher levels of oxygen absorption and lower heart rates than the athletes in the control group.

- Ginseng helps the blood vessels in the lungs absorb oxygen and circulate this oxygen-rich blood throughout the body. Studies done at the University of Munich in Germany show that regular use of ginseng increases the body's oxygen absorption, which is the actual measure of a person's aerobic capacity. (A person's actual aerobic capacity is not a measure of how much oxygen the lungs can hold but how much oxygen the body can absorb and utilize.)

• Ginseng improves cardiovascular conditioning. Athletes who took ginseng for nine weeks had a lower heart rate during intense exercise than athletes given placebos. This performance-enhancing benefit didn't show up for two months.

While the precise mechanism is not fully understood, researchers believe that ginseng offers these sports-enhancing benefits by increasing the production of the hormone corticosterone by the body's adrenal glands. In the body, this hormone causes the liver and muscles to make and store glycogen from the carbohydrates we eat; this glycogen is then converted to sugar for energy during exercise. Corticosterone helps the body use glycogen efficiently. It also balances the levels of potassium and sodium in the cells.

Ginseng also encourages the production, use, and storage of adenosine triphosphate (ATP), an enzyme that helps the muscles store fuel. In one study of 150 herbs, ginseng stimulated the production of ATP more than any other.

Ginseng's sports-enhancing benefits have been shown to continue after users cool down and leave the locker room. After a strenuous workout, ginseng can help the body recover faster. In one study, thirty people took ginseng for several months, and all but one reported that they recovered faster after a challenging workout than they did before taking the herb.

If a person overdoes it during a workout, ginseng can help prevent overworked muscles from cramping and growing stiff by lowering the amount of lactic acid in the blood. The body forms lactic acid when the muscles burn glycogen for energy; researchers measure physical fatigue by measuring how much lactate (a salt derived from lactic acid) is in the blood. The body needs oxygen to convert extra lactic acid back into glycogen; if this conversion back to glycogen does not occur, the lactic acid lingers in the muscles and makes them cramp. Researchers measure physical fatigue by measuring lactic acid by-products in the blood; the lower the levels of lactic acid in the body, the higher the level of overall fitness.

Researchers at the Institute for the Prophylaxis of Circulatory Diseases at the University of Munich in Germany gave ginseng extract to athletes, then measured their lactic acid levels before and after exercise. After nine weeks, the athletes' average lactate level was just half what it had been at the start of the experiment, indicating improved endurance. Another benefit of lowering lactic acid levels by taking ginseng: People are apt to experience less pain and stiffness when their muscles are overworked.

HOW GOOD IS THE SCIENCE?

Ginseng has been used as a healing herb for thousands of years, but only recently has it gone under the microscope of modern science. While thousands of studies have been done on ginseng and related herbs, many of these studies falls short of modern standards of "good science."

There are a number of problems with the studies. For one thing, a great deal of the research on ginseng has been conducted in Chinese and not translated into English. While many of the findings may be relevant to Western scientists, the language barrier has prevented the information from reaching a wider audience.

Another problem is that much of the research has not been done on whole ginseng plants but rather on ginseng extracts or individual ginsenosides. Perhaps some qualities of the whole plant do not show up in studies of its individual components.

Most studies have been done using animals, animal cell cultures, or human cell cultures rather than humans. While animal and laboratory research can reveal interesting findings, the most accurate information on an herb's effectiveness depends on its use in human subjects. In order to determine the actual efficacy of ginseng, researchers need to do studies involving whole plants in human subjects.

Of the studies that have been done using human volunteers, many did not include a control group. For a study to be considered reliable, it must compare people receiving treatment with those in the same circumstances who do not receive treatment. Only by comparing the two groups (without the researchers or the participants knowing who is receiving the actual treatment and who is receiving a placebo or dummy treatment) can a study reflect accurate, unbiased results. These studies are known as double-blind studies because neither the researchers nor the study participants know who received the treatment.

The conclusion: Ginseng is one of the most widely used herbs in the world, but few well-controlled studies have been done on it. The experience of millions of people over thousands of years provides compelling evidence of ginseng's effectiveness, but the chances are good that the herb will not gain respect among most Western doctors until more well-designed studies are done to document its effectiveness.

CHAPTER 5

Ginseng and Stress

Ironically, the very herb that can boost your energy level in times of fatigue can also calm your nerves in times of stress. Ginseng has sedative properties that make it useful when facing the challenges of a difficult relationship, a high-pressure job, an uncomfortable social setting, or any other stressful situation. Ginseng can help you face stressful events without experiencing the physiological changes that can cause you to feel overcome by the unpleasant side effects of stress.

Unchecked, stress can be hazardous to your health. Life can be stressful, and stress can be dangerous to the body. Stress contributes to high blood pressure, cardiovascular disease, digestive troubles, gastric ulcers, fatigue, insomnia, impotence, migraine headaches, memory problems, cancer, and weakened resistance to other diseases as well. Fortunately, ginseng can help you cope with stress, tension, and anxiety.

THE BODY UNDER STRESS

Stress is unavoidable; it is a part of being alive. Some people can cope with stress better than others. Your attitudes, expectations, perceptions, and personality have a lot to do with how you handle stress and how your body reacts to it.

When the body perceives stress, it kicks into the so-called fight-or-flight response, which involves a number of biochemical changes that occur in preparation for dealing with danger. In evolutionary terms, this high-intensity state makes sense because quick bursts of energy were required to fight off predators or flee a dangerous situation. Of course, in our daily lives we face fewer of these life-or-death threats, but the modern world remains full of stressors—financial worries, subways, children, health concerns, deadline pressures, relationship problems. When confronted with these stressors, our bodies respond in much the same way as our prehistoric ancestors once did. Much of the stress we experience in our daily lives cannot be managed by either fighting or fleeing. Therefore, all too often we respond to stress by internalizing our emotions and suppressing our anger, fear, or other feelings. Despite the circumstances, our body has entered a state of high-stress preparedness.

In the body, any stressor—either real or imagined—triggers an alarm in the hypothalamus in the midbrain. The hypothalamus then shifts into overdrive, warning the body that it must prepare for an emergency. As a result, the heart races, breathing speeds up, muscles tense, metabolism kicks into high gear, and blood pressure soars. Blood concentrates in the muscles, leaving hands and feet cold and muscles ready for action. Senses become more acute: Hearing becomes sharper and pupils dilate. The body is ready to fight or flee.

As part of the intricate system of stress responses, the body also releases adrenaline, epinephrine, cortisol, and other chemicals that inhibit the immune system and interfere with digestion, reproduction, growth, and tissue repair. While not harmful in short bursts, these responses can cause serious health problems if the stress continues for long periods of time. For example, someone working in a high-stress job, going through a difficult divorce, or recovering from abuse as a child might experience physiological effects of stress, such as menstrual cycle irregularity or an ulcer.

Over the long haul, these stress responses can contribute to the development of disease. Chronic stress can elevate blood pressure, contributing to hypertension; it can cause muscle tension, resulting in headaches and digestive disorders; it can suppress the immune system, leaving the individual prone to colds, flu, and a range of serious diseases. Stress can cause a number of specific illnesses, such as depression, irritable bowel syndrome, and other gastrointestinal disorders. A study done by the

U.S. Department of Health and Human Services Epidemiology Center in Atlanta, Georgia, found that during periods of national economic instability or recession, there was a marked increase in the number of people who experienced peptic ulcers, heart attacks, impotence, and weight loss, to name a few.

Because of the harmful effects of stress, it is essential to control stress and minimize the harm it causes in your body. The wise use of ginseng can help you cope with stress and minimize the damage it can cause.

CONSIDER THE EVIDENCE

A number of studies have demonstrated the sedative properties of ginseng. The following section describes how ginseng can be used to reduce overall stress, to improve alertness, and to enhance mental performance. Ginseng improves the body's ability to function under physical or mental stress. It improves blood flow to the brain, improving concentration and mental performance even when the body is under stress. Consider the results of these important studies:

GINSENG AND STRESS

Ginseng can calm the body and relieve stress without causing feelings of fatigue or grogginess. Literally hundreds of experiments have shown that ginseng can improve the body's performance under physical and mental stress. Here are a few of the highlights.

- A number of studies done in laboratories in Bulgaria, England, Korea, Russia, and the United States have shown that ginseng helps mice tolerate stressful situations. After taking ginseng, the mice were better able to "absorb stress" without experiencing distress or abnormal behavior. Animals that took ginseng not only coped better with stress but their body activity settled back to normal more quickly. In other words, the ginseng increased the animal's resistance to stress. This calming effect may explain why Chinese soldiers have been known to take ginseng with them into battle.

- One study done at the University of London explored the role of ginseng's impact on stress. For the study, researchers gave ginseng extract to one group of laboratory mice and a placebo to another group. The researchers then put the mice into a stressful situation—on a large white disk under a bright light. The researchers found that they could not distinguish the difference in behavior between the mice on ginseng and those not receiving the herb during normal daily activities, but under stress the mice given ginseng were much more able to respond well to the stress.

- Ginseng has been shown to help the body adapt to extreme temperatures. In one study, 1,000 workers at a polar station in the Arctic region were given ginseng for five months. Over the period of one year, there was a 40 percent reduction in the number of days lost from work and a 50 percent drop in overall sickness, compared to the previous year.

- In another study, 1,200 workers at a car factory in the Soviet Union were given ginseng in the spring and fall for two years. The rate of illness dropped by 20 percent compared to a similar group of workers who did not receive the herb. The same study showed that although an equal number of participants began the study with high blood pressure, by study's end the group that did not take ginseng contained three and a half times more people with high blood pressure.

GINSENG AND ALERTNESS

If you've ever been startled by a ringing phone in the middle of the night, you know that there is a direct link between stress and alertness or wakefulness. While intense bursts of stimulation can jolt the brain and bring it to attention, prolonged exposure to intense stimulation can leave a person feeling exhausted and unfocused.

In terms of brain chemistry, the initial stimulation triggers the release of a surge of adrenaline, creating the classic feelings of fight or flight. If the stimulation continues either due to an excessively stimulating environment or to prolonged stress or anxiety, the adrenal glands continue to pump out stress hormones known as corticosteroids. These hormones circulate to the brain and throughout the body, making the body feel alert, motivated, and eager to act.

- Ginseng helps to encourage feelings of alertness without harmful side effects. Researchers have given ginseng to fatigued mice attempting to maneuver a maze and fatigued people attempting to communicate using Morse code; in both experiments, the participants taking ginseng were better able to meet the mental challenge with improved focus and mental acuity. Ginseng also achieves this state of alertness without the harmful side effects associated with other stimulants.

- A study done at the University of London showed that ginseng actually increased the amount of corticosteroids reaching the brain. The researchers gave animals measured amounts of ginseng and hormones, and found that much more of the hormones reached the brains of the animals taking ginseng. Thus, individuals who take ginseng can experience the alertness and readiness to meet challenges without their bodies being flooded with high levels of stress hormones.

- Researchers from the University of Japan have found that ginseng helps to regulate the hypothalamus and pituitary glands in the brain. These parts of the brain actually communicate directly with the adrenal glands, telling them to send out stress hormones. Ginseng allows the brain to achieve the desired state of arousal with a minimal release of stress hormones.

GINSENG AND MENTAL PERFORMANCE

Ginseng appears to improve mental functioning by increasing blood flow to the brain. Ginseng allows the body to adjust or adapt to stress, without negative side effects. A number of studies have shown the ginseng use correlates with reduced stress, and improved mental performance.

- In one study, forty-five people with limited blood flow to the brain were given the prescription drug Hydergin (a drug commonly used to treat the problem), a ginseng extract, or a placebo. The ginseng extract improved blood flow to the brain by 34 percent, compared with 58 percent for the Hydergin group, and less than 1 percent for the placebo group.

- In another study, two hundred people also suffering from limited blood flow to the brain due to arteriosclerosis were given either 500 milligrams of standardized ginseng extract or a placebo. Fully 36 percent of the people receiving ginseng had "very favorable" improvement in blood flow and 54 percent had small improvements in the elasticity of the arteries and in blood flow; only 10 percent did not benefit from the ginseng. These studies may support and explain what the Chinese knew thousands of years ago: Ginseng is an excellent daily supplement for elderly people.

KEEPING THE BALANCE: GINSENG AS AN ADAPTOGEN

Unlike other herbs that tend to be either stimulating or sedating, ginseng is an adaptogen, or an agent that helps to keep the body in balance. The word "adaptogen" comes from the Greek words *adapto*, meaning "to adjust," and -*gen*, meaning "producing." It was coined by the Soviet scientist N. V. Lazarev in 1974. Adaptogens help the body adjust to stress and maintain balance.

Many Western researchers have trouble accepting the concept of adaptogens because they tend to view the body as a series of isolated systems rather than as an interconnected whole. Western healers tend to think every health problem has a specific cause and cure (usually a drug to alleviate a given symptom or complaint). Eastern healers, on the other hand, traditionally view the body in holistic terms, acknowledging complex interactions that create overall physical health and spiritual well-being. When it comes to managing stress, ginseng and other adaptogens help the body remain balanced both hormonally and emotionally.

According to researchers, in order to be considered an adaptogen, an herb must: (1) not harm or disrupt the body; (2) act in a nonspecific way; and (3) bring the body back into balance, whether the pathology being treated involves a state of excess or inadequacy. Adaptogens, including ginseng, are believed to strengthen the body in several key ways. For example, they:

- Bolster the adrenal glands
- Allow the cells to utilize more energy
- Encourage the elimination of toxins at the cellular level
- Help the body use oxygen more effectively
- Strengthen the body's biorhythms

Ginseng is considered an ideal example of an adaptogen, as it is effective at both energizing the body and calming it down, depending on the needs of the individual. Researchers have attempted to demonstrate ginseng's adapotenic properties. In various studies, mice have been exposed to toxins (including drugs used in chemotherapy), to infectious bacteria, and to extremes in heat and cold and changes in air pressure. In each of the studies, the mice given ginseng were better able to combat stress, but the same mice did not show any changes if they received ginseng when they were not under stress. In other words, the ginseng helped equalize or normalize the animal's body, but it did not overcorrect or act in only one direction. Taken together, these studies demonstrate ginseng's effectiveness as an adaptogen.

While researchers have been able to demonstrate ginseng's behavior as an adaptogen, they cannot fully explain how it works. Ginseng seems to have an effect on the hormones, specifically its ability to make the hormone messenger systems more effective. By facilitating better communication among the body's defenses, ginseng may help to correct a number of problems by bringing the body back into balance. By encouraging balance rather than a specific physical response, ginseng can normalize blood pressure by raising or lowering blood pressure as needed.

Ginseng may perform its balancing act by strengthening the adrenal glands. It seems to play a role in the regulation of the levels of the hormone ACTH (adrenocorticotropic hormone) in the blood, which in turn stimulates adrenal activity. As an adaptogen, ginseng may fine-tune the levels of ACTH and adrenaline based on an individual's specific needs. It increases the energy levels in those who are losing steam, and it calms or sedates those who feel anxious and over-excited.

Researchers have examined the role of the adrenal glands in stress. In one experiment, researchers removed the adrenal glands of laboratory rats to eliminate the possibility of natural production of stress hormones. The animals were divided into two groups, and half were given ginseng for eight days while the others received a placebo. The rats were then injected with the stress hormone corticosterone. The researchers found that up to seven times more corticosterone collected around the hypothalamus in the brain of the rats treated with ginseng, compared with those animals receiving a placebo. The hypothalamus strives to keep the stress hormones in balance, lowering stress hormone levels when they reach higher than normal levels. Ginseng appears to make the hypothalamus more effective at controlling stress.

Unfortunately, this biological process is not well understood. Some studies have shown the beneficial effects of ginseng even in mice that have had their adrenal glands removed. While ginseng may work on both the adrenal glands and the brain itself, the precise mechanism of ginseng still remains a mystery.

CHAPTER 6

Ginseng
and the Immune System

Your overall health depends on the ability of your immune system to fight off disease. The immune system is the way the body fights invaders, such as viruses, bacteria, and fungi that can cause diseases. These invaders can cause a range of health problems, from everyday complaints like the common cold to more serious conditions such as cancer, multiple sclerosis, asthma, Epstein-Barr syndrome, and chronic fatigue syndrome.

Your immune system can be compromised or weakened by emotional or physical stress, lack of sleep, poor diet, smoking, or alcohol consumption. Even pleasurable but intense experiences—such as going on a long vacation or starting a new job—can decrease your immune response, leaving you more vulnerable to disease.

While ginseng has long been known as a tonic herb that can improve overall health, researchers now know that it strengthens the body by strengthening the immune system. Because it makes the immune system stronger, ginseng helps the body respond to stressful situations without experiencing the physical problems associated with chronic stress. Researchers have shown that people under stress have weakened immunity, leaving them more susceptible to infections, circulatory disease, and other conditions thought to arise from inner imbalance.

UNDERSTANDING IMMUNITY

The immune system allows the body to coexist with hundreds of millions of bacteria and other microorganisms, but to remain ready to search out and destroy any of these cells when they threaten the body. Twenty-four hours a day, the immune system hunts down viruses, bacteria, and other potentially harmful cells.

The immune system consists of three different integrated systems—the barriers, the non-specific defenses, and the specific defenses.

THE BARRIERS

In order for pathogens to enter the body, they must break through the body's physical barriers. One of the most important (and most obvious) of the barriers is the skin, which consists of seven layers of tightly packed cells glued together with an intercellular cement. The mucous membranes are specialized skin cells that release sticky fluids to trap pathogens and wash them out of the body. These secretions include nasal mucus, saliva, stomach acid, digestive juices, tears, urine, vaginal secretions, prostate secretions, and the oily secretion of the skin and scalp. Many of these secretions contain special properties; for example, the stomach acid, urine, and reproductive secretions contain acids that can kill some microorganisms. In addition, the oily secretions of the skin, tears, and saliva contain antibiotic-like substances.

The barrier system also includes an essential secretion known as hyaluronic acid. This is a mucus-like connective tissue that bathes and nourishes each cell; its gelatinous texture helps hold the cells of the body in place. This extracellular fluid makes up about one-fifth of the liquid of the body. It allows the transfer of nutrients, waste materials, and other chemicals between the tiny blood vessels known as capillaries and the individual cells themselves, and between the lymphatic system and the cells.

The viscosity or thickness of the fluid is determined by two main components, hyaluronic acid, which is secreted by the connective tissues, and hyaluronidase, an enzyme that thins the secretion to the appropriate consistency. If these two components fall out of balance, the fluid will become too thick or too thin. Some bacteria and viruses contain hyaluronidase so that they can thin or "melt" the fluid and work their way through their barrier; when the immune system is healthy, the fluid is thick enough that it is difficult or impossible for pathogens to enter the body.

THE NON-SPECIFIC DEFENSES

The non-specific defenses respond to any particle or pathogen that can't be recognized as "friendly." The non-specific defenses alert the specific defenses that a pathogen has entered the body, and the specific defenses then search and destroy their target. There are several types of non-specific defenses. The body has specialized defense cells, including phagocytes (the most important of the non-specific defenses) and natural killer cells (discussed on page 96).

In addition, the body defends itself through the physiological responses of inflammation and fever. Inflammation prevents the spread of the microorganisms further into the body, it increases the circulation of white blood cells and immune cells to the damaged tissues, and it helps the body remove the dead cells to promote tissue healing. Fever is part of the immune response because some pathogens cannot survive the elevated temperatures.

The body also contains its own set of disinfectant chemicals. These chemicals, which are present in the blood and extracellular fluid, kill bacteria and support the immune system by starting inflammation. Other chemicals, such as interferon, help the body prevent a virus from infecting other cells.

THE SPECIFIC DEFENSES

Each of the specific defense mechanisms—the antibodies, lymphocytes, plasma cells, and T-cells—has specialized capabilities and each is designed to counter a specific antigen. Antigens are proteins present in bacteria, viruses, and other particles that are foreign to the human body.

The specific defense cells have several special characteristics. They work throughout the entire body, rather than simply at the site of the infection. They have the power to clone themselves as many times as they need to defeat an invader. They also remember the invading pathogen so that they can wage an even bigger defense if it should ever return. (Cell memory is what allows immunizations to be effective.)

With this basic understanding of how the immune system works, you can better appreciate the ways that ginseng helps to strengthen the immune system. The following section presents some of the evidence of how ginseng enhances the immune system.

CONSIDER THE EVIDENCE

A number of studies have demonstrated the immune-enhancing properties of ginseng.

- Ginseng has been shown to increase the number of infection-fighting natural killer (NK) cells and white blood cells. Blood samples analyzed after one month of regular ginseng use showed a range of positive effects; the immune-enhancing benefits were even greater after two months.

- In one landmark study, conducted from 1975 to 1980, more than 60,000 workers at the Volzhsky car factory in the Soviet Union were given extract of Siberian ginseng daily for several months. The workers' overall health improved and they missed fewer days of work. Similar studies with other types of ginseng have been done on long-distance Soviet truck drivers, also with impressive results.

- Ginseng can boost immunity and improve resistance to disease. Animals given ginseng and then infected with disease-causing bacteria were found to be less likely to become sick than others.

- In Japan, researchers have found that ginseng can boost the immune system by increasing the number of protective white blood cells and antibodies that work as the first line of defense against disease.

- Studies conducted at the Central Drug Research Laboratory in Lucknow, India, suggest that several types of ginseng may even be able to stimulate the body to produce more interferon, the antiviral protective protein.

- Research done at the Department of Pharmacology at the University of Milan, Italy, has found that healthy people, after taking ginseng for eight weeks, had a more powerful immune system that was capable of resisting harmful bacteria, cancer cells, and other unwanted guests in the body compared with those who took a placebo.

- Ginseng can be effective at combating the flu. A study conducted at the Department of Pharmacology at the University of Milan, Italy, in 1996, used a standardized extract of ginseng to increase the immune response. For twelve weeks, 227-volunteers took 100 milligrams of standardized ginseng or a placebo. Everyone received a flu shot at four weeks. In the weeks after the shot, 42 people in the placebo group developed flu or a cold, while just 15 people in the ginseng group became sick. Blood tests showed that antibody levels were signif-

BOX: NATURAL KILLER CELLS TO THE RESCUE

Natural killer cells play an essential part of the immune system by searching for and destroying cancer cells and viruses. Known more formally as cytotoxic T-cells, natural killer cells can be described as serial killers: They can attack one cell after another as long as they can find unwanted cells on which to feast.

icantly higher in the ginseng group, and levels of natural killer cells were almost twice as high in that group, compared to the placebo group.

- Ginseng helps the body resist colds and flu. In one study, truck drivers took Siberian ginseng extract with their tea for six years. During that time, the number of drivers who became sick from flu dropped from 41 per 1,000 to less than 3 per 1,000. The number of days lost per year due to illness dropped from 286 per 100 workers to 11 per 100.

GINSENG'S LIMITS

Despite its impressive record, even ginseng can't do it all. It doesn't work as an antibiotic; ginseng is ineffective in fighting bacteria, viruses, or any other infectious agent. Ginseng combats these conditions by strengthening immunity after it has been compromised by exhaustion, stress, or other situations that leave the body weakened.

As an immune enhancer, ginseng is very effective in situations involving convalescence. When the body is weak and infirm, ginseng helps to strengthen the immune system and boost energy levels. In these situations, ginseng does not cure any specific illness but rather helps the body regain its strength after a period of physical stress or illness.

When it comes to boosting immunity, don't rely on ginseng alone, although it may have a role in your overall health maintenance program. Ginseng should be only one part of your strategy for leading a good life, which should include a healthy lifestyle, a balanced diet, and other health-enhancing behaviors.

FOR MORE INFORMATION

If you would like more information about the immune system or immune system disorders, discuss the matter with your doctor and contact one or more of the following organizations:

American Auto Immune Related Diseases Association
Michigan National Bank Building
15475 Gratiot
Detroit, MI 48205
(313) 371-8600

Immune Deficiency Foundation
25 West Chesapeake Avenue
Towson, MD 21204
(410) 321-6647

GINSENG IN COMBINATION

Ginseng often is used with other herbs to enhance the immune system. A popular herbal formula used in China and Japan to strengthen the immune system is called Shosai koto. This formula has been shown to stop certain viruses and stop the growth of certain tumors. Shosai koto, which means "detailed things" in English, contains ginseng in combination with

- Licorice (*Glycerriza glabra*)

- Bupleurum (*Bupleurum falcatum*)

- Chinese skullcap (*Scutellaria baicalensis*)

Several other herbs have established reputations as immune enhancers. These include:

- Astragalus root (*Astragalus membranaceus*)

- Codonopsis root (*Condonopis piloula*)

- Echinacea root (*Echinacea purpurea and E. angustifolia*)

CHAPTER 7

Ginseng
and Sexual Function

Ginseng is an herb with a reputation: In cultures around the world, it is known and valued as an aphrodisiac and sexual aid. To some degree, ginseng earned this reputation based on the shape of the root. According to the ancient Chinese Doctrine of Signatures, a plant that physically resembled a part of the body was considered healing for that body part. Because ginseng root has a somewhat human form—including arms, legs, and sometimes phallic parts—the root has been credited with making men sexually potent, virile, and vigorous. As a result, many people consider ginseng to be very powerful at boosting sexual desire and performance.

According to Chinese lore, Chinese emperors used ginseng to boost their sexual energy, which was supposed to be a sign of the overall health and vitality of the empire. Chinese myth holds that one emperor actually parted with his entire fortune in order to obtain a well-endowed ginseng root, in hopes of improving his sexual performance.

While many Asian cultures appreciated the power of ginseng to enhance sexual function, they did not necessarily view ginseng as an aphrodisiac. Instead, the herb was considered a tonic, which could improve overall energy, including sexual energy. In many Asian cultures, sexual potency is seen as a measure of good overall health, so it comes as no surprise that stronger sexual urges were associated with the energizing effects of ginseng.

Ginseng's reputation as an aphrodisiac probably started when Europeans noted the herb's effect on sexual vitality. In this way, they may have confused overall energy and vitality with sexual energy and vitality. Chinese researchers have noted that ginseng does not "lead you to do things you would not do anyway" and that it "just strengthens you to do what is normal." In other words, ginseng won't unleash excessive sexual urges, but it can restore a diminished sexual drive.

In addition to its use in encouraging sexual function, ginseng is used to strengthen the reproductive system as a whole. In North America, the Native Americans used ginseng to promote fertility for both men and women. The Delaware and Mohegan tribes recommended it for numerous afflictions of the sexual organs, and the Cherokee believed it strengthened the womb.

CONSIDER THE EVIDENCE

Animals studies have found that ginseng may affect the reproductive hormones in certain important ways. In fact, some researchers have gone so far as to describe ginseng's effect on the body as gonadotropic, or one that stimulates the function of the gonads (sex glands). Impressed with these findings about ginseng's influence on sexuality, some farmers in the Soviet Union have used Siberian ginseng to stimulate animal breeding, especially among animals that showed signs of retarded growth or poor development.

Human studies on hormone levels and ginseng have been less conclusive. In most studies, researchers have not found changes in hormone levels after participants take ginseng. One explanation for these findings is that the people who participated in the study were all healthy, so perhaps they did not need their hormones changed. Remember, ginseng strives to balance the hormones and maintain harmony in the body. If this is true, then ginseng would be expected to increase the hormone levels of only those people who were experiencing a hormone deficiency.

Researchers suspect that if ginseng does affect hormones, it does so by stimulating the brain's hypothalamus and pituitary glands to alter the production of sex hormones; it also may make certain cells more or less receptive to hormones.

GINSENG AND IMPOTENCE

In the age of the anti-impotence drug Viagra, some people may see ginseng as a less preferable (and less dramatic) treatment for sexual dysfunction. However, ginseng offers a natural, safe, and successful way to manage impotence while at the same time improving overall energy and health.

Many men in Asian cultures have been known to suck on a ginseng root before intercourse to improve their satisfaction and performance. While there is no evidence to suggest that ginseng acts immediately to create arousal and to enhance performance, studies have shown that ginseng has a role in fine-tuning hormone levels and sexual function.

Impotence may be caused by physical problems. To achieve an erection, there must be cooperation among blood vessels, nerves, and tissues. A number of health problems—including circulatory problems, cardiovascular disease, diabetes, stroke, epilepsy, Alzheimer's disease, neurological disorders, alcohol and drug abuse, Parkinson's disease, and liver and kidney disease—can cause impotence. So can certain medications, including tranquilizers, diuretics, and anti-ulcer, antipsychotic, antidepressant, and antihypertensive drugs. Some over-the-counter antihistamines and decongestants can cause temporary impotence as well.

Ginseng may help to reverse impotence by boosting the hormones responsible for sexual response. Men experiencing impotence caused by physical factors, may experience a decline in hormones that control sexual response. Ginseng has been shown to contain certain compounds that affect the levels of sex hormones in the body; in fact, it actually can increase the levels of male sex hormones.

Many cases of impotence involve psychological problems or emotional difficulties with a partner. Ginseng will not help in these situations; the best course of action may be to discuss the matter with a counselor or other mental health professional.

- In many cases, ginseng has been used in Asian cultures to combat impotence, especially impotence that accompanies aging and a general lack of vitality and energy. Chinese healers often prescribe long-term use of ginseng to reinvigorate the body and to offset the natural decline in potency that is part of the aging process. Japanese and Korean hospitals have been using ginseng extracts for decades to treat impotence.

- Ginseng can be especially effective in people whose production of sex hormones has begun to decline due to age, stress, or illness. It can, however, be counterproductive in certain circumstances. Consider a young man at his sexual peak who uses ginseng to boost his sexual performance. Say he chose the strongest red Korean ginseng he could find in hopes of experiencing an exceptional sexual high. He would find that this stimulating, heating ginseng could actually impair his sexuality. Because he already has excess sexual energy, in order to balance his body he needs a more cooling or relaxing herb (perhaps American ginseng), not further stimulation.

- One study conducted at the Yonsei University College of Medicine in Seoul, Korea, looked at the efficacy of treating erectile dysfunction in ninety patients. While there wasn't complete remission of the problem, 60 percent of the men taking ginseng showed improvement, compared to only 30 percent of the men in the control group or those taking another drug to treat the problem (Trazodone).

- Russian researchers found that ginseng is effective in treating some cases of impotence. Dr. Brekhman, the leading Soviet ginseng researcher, gave ginseng to forty-four patients with impotence who had not responded to any other medications. Twenty-one of those patients recovered completely, and others improved. In another study, ginseng was given to twenty-seven impotent patients.

Fifteen recovered completely, and nine improved. In addition, the men taking ginseng felt more tranquil and active. Although much more study is needed, we can say that the Chinese may be justified in expecting to be sexually active in old age with the help of nothing more than ginseng.

Other herbs commonly used in combination with ginseng in the treatment of impotence include:

- Yohimbe bark (*Pausinystalia yohimbe*)
- Wild oats (*Avena sativum*)
- Ginkgo (*Ginkgo biloba*)
- Damiana leaves (*Turnea aphrodisiaca*)

FOR MORE INFORMATION

If you have a problem with impotence that does not respond to treatment with ginseng, consider contacting one of the following organizations for additional information:

American Association of Sex Educators, Counselors and Therapists
435 North Michigan Avenue, Suite 1717
Chicago, IL 60611
(312) 644-0828

Impotence Information Center
American Medical Systems
Minneapolis, MN 55440
(800) 543-9632

Impotence Institute of America
10400 Little Patuxent Parkway, Suite 485
Columbia, MD 21044
(410) 715-9605

Potency Restored
8630 Fenton Street, Suite 218
Silver Spring, MD 20910
(301) 588-5777

GINSENG, INFERTILITY, AND SEX HORMONES

Ginseng also may enhance male fertility. Ginseng stimulates the adrenal glands, encouraging the production of testosterone, as well as estrogen and progesterone.

- A 1996 study published in an Italian medical journal reported that sixty-six patients were treated either with ginseng or a placebo. Those using the ginseng showed an increase in the number of sperm and an improvement in sperm motility after taking the herb.

- In studies quoted by the Ginseng Research Institute in Wausau, Wisconsin, it was concluded that ginseng indirectly helps men who do not have sufficient sex hormones. Studies done in China indicate that ginseng increases the sperm's motility and raises the sperm count in men who have low numbers.

- Much of the research done on hormone

111

levels has been performed on laboratory animals. Researchers have found that ginseng increases the sex hormones in rats and rabbits and that, at high doses, it is a uterine toner. It also increases the male hormone testosterone and increases the weight of the male sex organs in male rats; these ginseng-taking rats also have more sex than those not taking the herb. Ginseng offers special benefits to females; it increases the levels of the hormone prolactin, which then triggers an increase in progesterone levels, decreasing the potentially harmful effects of excess estrogen in the body.

- In one experiment, ginseng glycosides encouraged development of sex organs in young animals. Young male mice given ginseng reached puberty faster than untreated mice, and their prostate glands were 40 to 60 percent larger. In some experiments the weight of the prostate gland and seminal vessels increased after taking ginseng.

GINSENG AND PREGNANCY

In China, ginseng has a long history of use during pregnancy. Ancient wisdom holds that ginseng can supply extra energy to both mother and baby if the herb is taken during pregnancy.

To date, only one well-controlled study has been published on the use of ginseng during pregnancy. As part of a 1991 study of 88 pregnant women in China, those taking ginseng experienced less pre-eclampsia (a complication of pregnancy involving high blood pressure) than those who did not take the herb. None of the women reported negative side effects associated with the ginseng use.

Although no negative side effects have been associated with the use of ginseng during pregnancy, you should discuss the matter with your obstetrician or health care provider before taking ginseng or any other herb during pregnancy. As always, you should not exceed the recommended dose and you should discontinue using ginseng if you experience high blood pressure. Korean and Asian red ginseng should be avoided because they are considered too stimulating during pregnancy. Also keep in mind that ginseng should not be used in combination with caffeine and other stimulants, especially during pregnancy.

FOR MORE INFORMATION

If you would like more information about the use of ginseng during pregnancy, discuss the matter with your doctor. For information on the ginseng and its safe use, contact one of the herbal organizations listed on pages 225-233. For information about pregnancy, consider contacting one of the following organizations.

American Board of Obstetrics and Gynecology
2915 Vine Street
Dallas, TX 75204
(214) 871-1619

American College of Nurse–Midwives
818 Connecticut Ave., NW
Suite 900
Washington, DC 20006
(202) 289-0171

Center for Humane Options in Childbirth Experience
3474 North High Street
Columbus, OH 43214
(614) 263-2229

National Women's Health Resource Center
2440 M Street, NW
Suite 325
Washington, DC 20037
(202) 293-6045

GINSENG AND MENOPAUSE

One out of every two women experiences some symptoms associated with menopause, and about one in four finds these physical changes uncomfortable to distressing. While some women experience increased energy and enthusiasm for life during menopause, most women have certain complaints, including the following:

- Hot flashes and sweating
- Facial flushing
- Vaginal dryness
- Headaches
- Heart palpitations
- Irregular periods
- Joint pain
- Depression
- Anxiety
- Irritability
- Lack of concentration

- Mood swings
- Sleep disturbances
- Forgetfulness

Ginseng relieves many menopausal complaints, a fact that has been supported by several studies with large groups of women.

- In one German study, for example, over half of the seventy-two menopausal women given ginseng found that all their symptoms—hot flashes, night sweats, nervous tension, headaches, and heart palpitations—completely disappeared when they took ginseng. In comparison, only 19 percent of women receiving the placebos experienced a decrease in symptoms. The women taking ginseng also experienced less depression and insomnia and fewer sexual problems. R. T. Own, M.D., the gynecologist who performed this study, suggests that women should take ginseng well before menopause begins, in order to prevent the symptoms from starting. Dr. Own adds, "If they receive this safe geriatric treatment regularly over a longer time, they will not require hormones."

- In a clinical trial, ginseng powder was given to eighty-three menopausal women for eight weeks. The symptoms of menopause—hot flashes, weakneess, and fatigue—were alleviated in fully 70 percent of the women.

- Ginseng is especially effective for hot flashes, and often completely eliminates them within six weeks. Robert Atkins, M.D., a well-known author and doctor of nutritional medicine, agrees. He found that out of hundreds of patients who complained about having hot flashes, about 80 percent responded to ginseng. The few women who do not get results from ginseng alone did so once vitamin E was added to their regimen. Many herbalists have noticed that vitamin E does seem to enhance the actions of herbs such as ginseng.

Other herbs considered effective in the treatment of menopausal symptoms include the following:

- Black cohosh root (*Cimicifuga rasemosa*)
- Vitex berry (*Vitex agnus castus*)
- Licorice root (*Glycyrrhiza glabra*)
- Dong quai root (*Angelica sinensis*)
- Motherwort leaves (*Leonorus cardiaca*)
- Fenugreek seed (*Trigonella foenumgrae-cum*)
- Evening Primrose oil (omega-6 fatty acids)

FOR MORE INFORMATION

If you experience unpleasant symptoms of menopause that do not respond to treatment with ginseng, consider requesting additional information about menopause from your doctor or from one of the following organizations:

American Menopause Foundation
Madison Square Station
P.O. Box 2013
New York, NY 10010
(212) 475-3107

North American Menopause Society
c/o University Hospitals of Cleveland
Dept. OB/GYN
Room 7024
1110 Euclid Avenue
Cleveland, OH 44106
(216) 844-8748

Society for Menstrual Cycle Research
10559 North 104th Place
Scottsdale, AZ 85258
(602) 451-9731

CHAPTER 8

Other Uses of Ginseng

Ginseng will not cure any specific disease or relieve any specific symptoms. It can't cure cancer, reverse aging, or eliminate the need for diabetes treatment. What ginseng can do is to improve your overall health, which in turn can help the body resist a number of illnesses or medical conditions, especially those associated with excessive stress.

While this may seem like a vague promise, the benefits can be significant. Consider that about 10 percent of Americans suffer from high blood pressure and other circulatory problems that can be triggered by anxiety and tension. Lowering tension and stress may in turn lower blood pressure among these people. In addition, stress can increase the cancer risk in humans. Stress also can cause people to be more susceptible to viral infections, such as cold and flu.

Ginseng improves overall health by working holistically. Unlike traditional pharmaceutical drugs, which work on a particular symptom or part of the body, ginseng works on the entire body. Most Western drugs weaken the body's overall system and diminish vitality while controlling symptoms, but ginseng and other tonic herbs strengthen the body's systems and in turn help to control symptoms.

But ginseng can't do it all. The best way to control physical deficiencies is to change the lifestyle patterns that cause the problems. The herbal approach to healing requires a holistic approach to health. No herb or herbal formula can correct significant health problems if the person also does not make appropriate lifestyle changes. Taking ginseng cannot reverse the negative consequences of bad health habits, including poor diet, inadequate sleep, excessive stress, minimal exercise, bad mental attitudes, and other lifestyle factors.

Still, evidence indicates that ginseng can play an important role in health management, especially when it is part of an overall positive approach to health. The following section summarize some of the conditions that researchers have shown respond well to the use of ginseng.

ALCOHOLISM AND DRUG ABUSE

A number of studies have shown that ginseng can be helpful during detoxification from alcohol or drug abuse. It helps to relieve the fatigue and poor vitality associated with the ongoing use of alcohol or drugs, especially sedatives or tranquilizers.

Detoxification is a crucial step in freeing a person from addiction to alcohol or drugs, including illegal drugs, prescription medications, and over-the-counter drugs. Herbs, including ginseng, can be quite helpful in removing drug-related toxins from the body, especially during the first four to six weeks of sobriety.

- Studies have found that people recover more quickly from alcohol's effect when they are taking ginseng. The herb stimulates the production of two liver enzymes, alcohol dehydrogenase and aldehyde dehydrogenase, which help the body convert alcohol in the liver to a less toxic form. When healthy volunteers drank excessive amounts of alcohol (2.5 ounces of 50-proof vodka for every 140 pounds of bodyweight in forty-five minutes), the ginseng kept the blood-alcohol levels much lower than when the same people drank the alcohol without taking the ginseng. In fact, nearly three out of four participants had half the blood-alcohol level when taking ginseng as they had when they did not use the herb.

- Studies done in Europe have shown that ginseng can slightly improve chronic liver disease in elderly people whose livers have been damaged by the excessive use of alcohol or drugs. After using ginseng, their liver enzyme levels improved, even though the liver itself had been damaged.

- Preliminary research indicates that ginseng may be helpful in the prevention of addiction to morphine and other strong pain relievers used in a medical setting. Japanese researchers at Nagasaki University conducted a study designed to test the effect of ginseng on painkilling drugs, including morphine. They found that ginseng inhibited patients' tolerance to and dependence on morphine.

If you are planning to detoxify your body from the effects of drugs and /or alcohol, discuss the use of ginseng with your health care professional. The energizing effects of the herb can mask symptoms of fatigue that may be caused by liver damage, a condition that needs to be treated by a medical professional.

FOR MORE INFORMATION

For more information on the treatment of alcoholism and drug abuse, discuss the matter with your doctor or contact one or more of the following organizations:

Center for Substance Abuse Prevention
(800) 843-4971

Cocaine Anonymous
(800) COCAINE; (213) 559-5833

The Hazelden Foundation
(800) I-DO-CARE

Johnson Institute
(800) 231-5165; (800) 247-0484

Narcotics Anonymous
(800) 662-4357; (818) 780-3951

National Association of Alcoholism and Drug Abuse Counselors
(703) 920-4644

National Clearinghouse for Alcohol and Drug Information
(301) 468-2600

National Council on Alcoholism and Drug Dependence
(212) 206-6770

National Institute on Alcoholism and Drug Abuse
(800) 662-4357; (301) 443-4373

Rational Recovery
(916) 621-4374

Secular Organizations for Sobriety (SOS)
(716) 834-2922

AGING

Traditional Chinese healers have long believed that ginseng offers long-term health benefits: They believe the benefits of using the herb are cumulative and that, with regular use, ginseng can improve health and vitality while prolonging life itself. The ancient Chinese prescription for health: Take some ginseng every day to ward off the illnesses associated with old age and to encourage a long life.

As they age, many people develop Alzheimer's disease, dementia, and other conditions that can rob them of the precious knowledge of who they are. Some 4 million older Americans—including two out of every three nursing-home patients—suffer from Alzheimer's disease or dementia.

With Alzheimer's disease, the body malfunctions and gradually destroys the nerve cells in several key areas of the brain. As the disease progresses, the nerve fibers around the hippocampus—the brain's memory center—become crossed and knotted; these neurofibrillary tangles make it impossible to store or retrieve information. In addition to this internal short circuit, the brain also experiences a drop in the concentration of neurotransmitting chemicals, which further breaks down the body's communications network.

Dementia (or senile dementia) refers to general mental deterioration, including memory loss, moodiness, irritability, personality changes, childish behavior, difficulty communicating, and inability to concentrate. Alzheimer's disease is a type of dementia. Many practitioners of traditional Chinese medicine recommend that people begin taking regular doses of ginseng after age forty in order to ward off these types of mental impairment that can accompany old age.

Ginseng has a reputation for enhancing memory and mental functioning, especially among older people. Ancient Chinese herbalists often recommended the use of ginseng for the "benefit of understanding." In the same way, Native Americans in the Great Lakes region used ginseng as a tonic to improve mental functioning.

- Most people become more forgetful as they age; by age sixty-five, about one out of every ten North Americans has a memory-loss disorder, such as Alzheimer's disease or senile dementia. Fortunately, much of this memory loss is preventable. A study funded by the National Institute on Aging followed study participants for twenty-eight years; it found that many people do not experience mental or intellectual decline, even when they are well into their seventh decade. The study found that people turning sixty-five now tend to be more mentally alert than people of previous generations, probably due to improved nutrition and education.

- Ginseng appears to be most effective for those people who experience a gradual decline in their mental abilities as they age, when they are sick, when working under stress, or when not following the basic rules of a healthy lifestyle.

- Ginseng probably works its magic by increasing the flow of oxygen to the brain and by strengthening the adrenal glands so that they can manage the symptoms of anxiety and stress that can derail the brain. The brain consumes a great deal of oxygen using fully one-fifth of the total oxygen in the blood. Most memory problems associated with aging are a result of poor circulation caused by hardening of the arteries or arteriosclerosis. This condition results from the formation of fatty deposits along the arterial walls. Ginseng has been shown to reverse the memory problems associated with blood flow to the brain. For example, an Italian researcher found that people who did nothing other than take a tincture of ginseng increased the blood flow to their brains by 34 percent; the people in the control group had no significant improvement.

- In one study conducted in the Soviet Union, ginseng was given to rats in their drinking water every other day for 320 days. Treated animals lived an average of 21 percent longer—799 days, compared to 659 days for animals not given ginseng.

FOR MORE INFORMATION

If someone you care about has symptoms of Alzheimer's disease or dementia, discuss the matter with your doctor. In addition, you might want to contact one or more of the following organizations:

Alzheimer's Disease and Related Disorders Association
919 North Michigan Avenue, suite 1000
Chicago, IL 60611
(312) 335-8700; (800) 272-3900

Alzheimer's Disease Society
2 West 45th Street, Room 1703
New York, NY 10036
(212) 719-4744

Association for Alzheimer's and Related Diseases
170 East Lake Street, Suite 600
Chicago, IL 60601-5997
(800) 572-6037; (800) 621-0379

ANEMIA

If you feel tired all the time and get winded faster than you used to, you may be experiencing anemia, a condition in which the blood is deficient in either red blood cells or the iron-containing hemoglobin portion of those cells.

Red blood cells transport oxygen from the lungs to the tissues and exchange the oxygen for carbon dioxide. If your red blood cells aren't up to the job, your tissues aren't getting enough oxygen. Fatigue and weakness are inevitable when your muscles, brain, and heart are working under such a strain. You may even appear pale and washed out because your skin lacks oxygen-rich red blood. Iron supports the function of many enzymes involved in the production of energy. Low levels of iron can contribute to some forms of anemia. Ginseng has been used in China for centuries to increase iron levels and red blood cells in the blood.

Ginseng can help in the treatment of anemia.

- In one study, fifty patients who did not respond to traditional drugs used to treat anemia were given ginseng. Their red blood cell count improved they experienced less fatigue, and their overall health became stronger.

- Other studies have shown that ginseng can increase the levels of white blood cells and platelets, components of the blood that assist in clotting.

FOR MORE INFORMATION

A number of organizations can provide information to people with anemia and blood disorders. Discuss the matter with your doctor and consider contacting one or more of the following groups:

American Society of Hematology
1200 19th Street, N.W., Suite 3000
Washington, DC 20036
(202) 857-1118

Franconia Research Foundation
1902 Jefferson Street, #2
Eugene, OR 97405
(503) 687-4658

National Heart, Lung, and Blood Institute
Information Center
National Institutes of Health
(301) 251-1222

CANCER

Every day our bodies produce more than 500 billion new cells. Every once in a while an error occurs, and our bodies form defective cells. This can be the beginning of cancer.

Cancer develops when oncogenes (the genes that control cell growth) are transformed by a carcinogen, or cancer-causing agent. In most cases the immune system identifies and destroys these aberrant cells before they multiply. But when the system breaks down, these fast-growing cancer cells reproduce, forming a tumor and invading healthy tissue. These tumors rob the body of nutrients and interfere with the tasks performed by the healthy tissue.

Ginseng has been shown to help boost the immune system and consequently to help slow or stop the spread of certain cancers. While the herb cannot be said to fight cancer directly, it does strengthen the body and improve its ability to fight for itself.

- Ginseng may help reduce the size of some tumors. Ginseng caused a 33 to 50 percent reduction in tumor size in laboratory mice that were implanted with tumors.

- Studies conducted at the Korea Cancer Center Hospital in Seoul have shown that people who take ginseng regularly tend to have fewer cancers of the liver, lungs, mouth, ovaries, pancreas, and stomach. (Ginseng did not appear to help prevent cancers of the bladder, breast, cervix, or thyroid.) According to the study, the most effective forms of ginseng were fresh extracts, white ginseng powders, and red ginseng roots.

- Ginseng has been found to be effective in helping people to cope with the sometimes debilitating effects of chemotherapy and radiation in the treatment of cancer. A number of studies done in the Soviet Union and Korea have shown that ginseng can help cancer patients tolerate treatments with less nausea and tiredness. In fact, ginseng is used for this purpose regularly in Russia.

- Ginseng has been found to minimize the cellular damage caused by radiation. One study found that rats exposed to radiation damage lived twice as long when given ginseng. Ginseng actually has been found to protect the cells from damage by radiation exposure. In addition, when damage does occur, ginseng is believed to help speed the healing process.

- Research done at the Petrov Oncological Institute in the Soviet Union found that cancer patients could tolerate 50 percent more of their chemotherapy drugs before experiencing negative side effects when they were given Siberian ginseng along with their drugs and surgery treatments. In addition, those who received Siberian ginseng and had surgery lived five months longer than those who did not take the ginseng.

- In animal studies, ginseng has been found to increase resistance to cancer-causing agents. It also was found to increase the activity of natural killer (NK) cells, the white blood cells that are critical in the fight against tumors.

FOR MORE INFORMATION

A number of organizations can help support and provide information to people battling cancer. The following groups may be of interest:

American Cancer Society
1599 Clifton Road, N.E.
Atlanta, GA 30329
(404) 320-3333

American Institute for Cancer Research
1759 R Street, N.W.
Washington, DC 20009
(202) 328-7744

Cancer Care
1180 Avenue of the Americas
New York, NY 10036
(212) 221-3300

Cancer Information Service
NCI/NIH
Building 31
9000 Rockville Pike
Bethesda, MD 20892
(800) 4-CANCER

Make Today Count
P.O. Box 222
Osage Beach, MO 65065
(314) 346-6644

National Coalition for Cancer Survivorship
1010 Wayne Avenue, 5th Floor
Silver Spring, MD 20910
(301) 650-8868

People Against Cancer
604 East Street
P.O. Box 10
Otho, IA 50569-0010
(515) 972-4444

CANCER AND ALTERNATIVE MEDICINE

Atkins Center for Complementary Medicine
152 East 55th Street
New York, NY 10022
(212) 758-2110

Can Help
3111 Paradise Bay Road
Port Ludlow, WA 98365-9771
(206) 437-2291

Cancer Treatment Centers of America
Memorial Medical Center and Cancer Institute
8181 South Lewis Avenue
Tulsa, OK 74137
(800) FOR-HELP; (918) 496-5000

Winifred Conkling

Committee for Freedom of Choice in Medicine
1180 Walnut Avenue
Chula Vista, VA 91911
(619) 429-8200

FACT—Foundation for Advancement in Cancer Therapy
P.O. Box 1242
Old Chelsea Station
New York, NY 10113
(212) 741-2790

Simonton Cancer Center
P.O. Box 890
Pacific Palisades, CA 90272
(800) 459-3424

Valley Cancer Institute
12099 West Washington Boulevard,
Suite 304
Los Angeles, CA 90066
(800) 488-1370; (213) 398-0013

CARDIOVASCULAR DISEASE

Your heart and circulatory system feed every cell in your body with life-giving oxygen. The 12,400-mile network of arteries, veins, and blood vessels known as your circulatory system circulates blood from your heart to the farthest reaches of your body. But all too often the system fails. Heart attacks, atherosclerosis, congestive heart failure, strokes, and other circulatory diseases claim about 1 million lives a year. In addition, more than 63 million Americans live with some form of heart or blood vessel disease. Heart disease kills more people than any other single ailment.

A number of studies have shown that ginseng can be effective in treating circulatory problems. Ginseng is used both to raise low blood pressure and to lower high blood pressure. It may seem strange to think of a single agent changing the body in seemingly opposite ways, but this merely demonstrates the Eastern philosophy of healing, which takes for granted the fact that remedies can work in more than one direction. As an adaptogenic treatment, ginseng helps the body adapt to its environment—in some cases by raising blood pressure and in others by lowering it.

> **NOTE:** If you have high blood pressure or any other cardiovascular problem, discuss treatment with your health care professional before using ginseng or any other herb.

• Ginseng is used in Chinese hospitals in emergency treatment to restore blood pressure of people in shock, in those who have had a heart attack, and for those who have lost excessive amounts of blood. It is also used to reduce high blood pressure, although in these cases the herb is usually part of a more complex treatment including diet, exercise, and other lifestyle changes.

• Chinese hospitals use sanchi ginseng to relieve spasms and pain associated with angina. Studies have shown that ginseng reduces these symptoms by about half in the people who use it.

- Because prescription drugs used to treat high blood pressure can have many side effects, doctors in Europe and Asia often recommend a trial of ginseng before patients must turn to drugs.

- Researchers in China have given ginseng extracts to patients following open heart surgery. A 1994 study compared patients receiving the ginseng with those who did not; the researchers found that cardiac patients who received ginseng after surgery experienced better recovery and less tissue damage due to lack of oxygen.

- Ginseng helps to lower blood cholesterol and triglyceride levels. High levels of both can contribute to the formation of atherosclerosis, or hardening of the arteries. In clinical experiments, ginseng also was found to raise levels of HDL, or "good," cholesterol, which is credited with removing plaque from the arteries. As a secondary benefit, ginseng helped relieve the secondary symptoms of atherosclerosis, including numbness in the limbs, cold extremities, insomnia, and heart palpitations. (Because American ginseng is less arousing, it tends to be more effective at altering cholesterol levels than Asian ginseng.)

- Ginseng contains calcium channel blockers, which help to correct high blood pressure and irregular heartbeat. Calcium channel blockers affect the movement of calcium into the cells of the heart and blood vessels. They help to relax blood vessels and increase the supply, of blood and oxygen to the heart.

FOR MORE INFORMATION

If you would like to know more about cardiovascular disease, talk to your health care provider and contact one or more of the following organizations:

American Heart Association
7272 Greenville Avenue
Dallas, TX 75231
(214) 373-6300

Citizens for Public Action on Blood Pressure and Cholesterol
P.O. Box 30374
Bethesda, MD 20824
(301) 770-1711

International Atherosclerosis Society
6550 Fannin, No. 1423
Houston, TX 77030
(713) 790-4226

Mended Hearts
7272 Greenville Avenue
Dallas, TX 75231-4966
(214) 706-1442

National Heart Lung and Blood Institute
Information Center
National Institutes of Health
(301) 251-1222

National Heart Savers Association
9140 West Dodge Road
Omaha, NE 68114
(402) 398-1993

National Hypertension Association
324 East 30th Street
New York, NY 10016
(212) 889-3557

CHRONIC FATIGUE SYNDROME

Ginseng's energizing effects have been shown to be effective in the treatment of chronic fatigue syndrome, a disorder whose symptoms include reduced mental alertness, depression, lack of motivation, irritability, hostility, indifference, unsociability, uncooperative behavior, lack of personal hygiene, and lack of appetite. Physical symptoms also include recurrent sore throats, low-grade fever, headaches, muscle pain, and lymph node swelling. The cause of the illness is unknown, though some doctors believe it is due to infection with the Epstein-Barr virus. The herb may work by bolstering the immune system or through another, as yet unknown mechanism.

In a study conducted at the University of Buenos Aires in Argentina, fifty people were identified as having the symptoms of chronic fatigue syndrome. The study participants were given a placebo for two weeks; then they were given a ginseng extract for

Winifred Conkling

fifty-six days. The researchers found that the ginseng caused a significant improvement in many of the symptoms of the syndrome.

FOR MORE INFORMATION

If you would like to know more about chronic fatigue syndrome, discuss the matter with your doctor and contact one or more of the following organizations:

American Auto Immune Related Diseases Association
Michigan National Bank Building
15475 Gratiot
Detroit, MI 48205
(313) 371-8600

Immune Deficiency Foundation
25 West Chesapeake Avenue
Towson, MD 21204
(410) 321-6647

DIABETES

Ginseng's adaptogenic properties are demonstrated in its use in treating diabetes. Diabetes is a disease that impairs the body's ability to produce insulin and to metabolize sugar. Normally the pancreas regulates the delicate balance of sugar in the bloodstream. But the 14 million Americans with diabetes mellitus cannot properly convert food (especially sugar) into energy, either because their bodies do not produce enough insulin (a hormone produced in the pancreas to regular blood-sugar levels) or because their bodies don't use the insulin they do produce properly. Instead, diabetics must monitor their blood-sugar levels, adjusting their diet and exercise—or their oral medications and insulin injections—to meet these changing conditions.

Diabetes can be difficult to detect. In fact, only about half of all diabetics know they have the disease. The symptoms of Type I insulin dependent diabetes—excessive thirst, frequent urination, dry mouth, blurred vision, and frequent infections—often develop rapidly. The signs of Type II diabetes—thirst, drowsiness, obesity, fatigue, tingling or numbness in the extremities, blurred vision, and itching—often go unrecognized for years before being properly diagnosed. Type I is sometimes called juvenile diabetes because it usually starts in childhood or early adulthood.

Ginseng's ability to stabilize blood-sugar levels has been known for centuries. As early as the first century A.D., Chinese healers used ginseng to reduce fatigue, excessive thirst, and frequent urination—classic signs of diabetes. In more recent history, ginseng was used by Japanese physicians to treat diabetes before insulin was available in the 1920s.

- In animal studies, ginseng has been shown to lower blood-sugar levels in animals that had their blood-sugar levels raised by ingesting excess sugar, and it also has been found to raise blood-sugar levels in animals that have had their levels artificially lowered by insulin injections.

- Dozens of clinical studies support the use of ginseng in treating diabetes. Several studies done in China show that ginseng lowers blood-sugar levels by 40 to 50 percent, sometimes eliminating the need for supplemental insulin. The levels remained low for a week or two after the ginseng was discontinued. As an added bonus, diabetics taking ginseng tend to have more energy, and those who experience impotence often find that the condition reverses itself.

- A study published in 1995 in the journal *Diabetes Care* concluded that ginseng may be a useful part of treatment for non–insulin-dependent diabetics. As part of a Finnish study, thirty-six patients were treated with ginseng or a placebo. The researchers found that the people taking 200 milligrams of ginseng experienced an improvement in mood and a reduced fasting blood glucose level.

- Diabetics who are resistant to insulin have been able to reduce the amount they take when they use ginseng as a supplement. In a study involving twenty-one patients with Type II diabetes, more than half improved after taking large daily doses (2,700 milligrams) of Korean red ginseng. After taking ginseng for about two months, blood-sugar levels of the Type II diabetics who were not taking insulin also dropped. No one in the study reported negative side effects.

- Japanese researchers at hospitals in Tokyo and Osaka gave diabetics capsules of ginseng with vitamin E. The treatment helped with complications from diabetes caused by poor circulation, nerve and kidney damage, impotence, and vision problems. The optimal dose as part of the treatment was 600 milligrams a day in the early treatment and 300 milligrams as a maintenance dose.

NOTE: If you're interested in using ginseng or any other herbs as part of the treatment of diabetes, you should discuss the matter with the doctor overseeing your condition.

FOR MORE INFORMATION

If you would like to know more about diabetes, discuss the matter with your primary care physician and contact one or more of the following organizations:

American Diabetes Association
National Center
P.O. Box 25757
1660 Duke Street
Alexandria, VA 22314
(703) 549-1500

Diabetes Research Institute Foundation
3440 Hollywood Boulevard, Suite 100
Hollywood, FL 33021
(305) 964-4040

International Diabetes Center
3800 Park Nicollet Boulevard
Minneapolis, MN 55416
(612) 927-3393

Joslin Diabetes Center
One Joslin Place
Boston, MA 02215
(617) 732-2415

HEARING AND VISION

A number of studies have found that ginseng can help to improve both hearing and vision among people with impaired senses. Once again, improved circulation appears to be one of the major reasons for the sensory enhancement.

- Researchers in the Soviet Union conducted more than sixty tests on the effect of Siberian ginseng on vision. They found that ginseng makes the eyes more responsive to light and better able to see in the dark.

- Ginseng also appears to protect the ears from damage due to loud noises. In one study, researchers examined the hearing of boat crew members who were surrounded by loud and incessant noise. During the study, the workers' hearing tolerance improved by two to four decibels and their inner ears were less traumatized than usual. The men in the control group who received a placebo instead of ginseng did not show any signs of improvement.

FOR MORE INFORMATION

If you would like more information on hearing or vision loss, discuss the matter with your doctor and contact one or more of the following organizations.

HEARING

American Speech-Language-Hearing Association
10801 Rockville Pike
Rockville, MD 20852
(301) 897-5700
(800) 638-8255

Better Hearing Institute
5021-B Backlick Road
Annandale, VA 22003
(800) EAR-WELL

International Hearing Society
20361 Middlebelt Road
Livonia, MI 48152
(810) 478-2610

National Institute on Deafness and Other Communication Disorders Clearinghouse
1 Communication Avenue

Bethesda, MD 20892-3456
(800) 241-1044
(800) 241-1055 (TDD)

SHHH (Self Help for Hard of Hearing People, Inc.)
7910 Woodmont Avenue, Suite 1200
Bethesda, MD 20814
(301) 657-2248
(301) 657-2249 (TTD)

For free information on hearing problems or a free over-the-phone hearing test, call Hearing Services at:

(800) 222-EARS
(800) 345-EARS (in Pennsylvania)

VISION

American Academy of Ophthalmology
655 Beach Street
San Francisco, CA 94109
(415) 561-8500

American Foundation for Vision Awareness
243 North Lindbergh Boulevard
St. Louis, MO 63141
(800) 927-2382

National Eye Institute
Building 31, Room 6-A32
31 Center Drive
MSC-2510
Bethesda, MD 20892-2510
(301) 496-5248

MENTAL HEALTH

Ginseng has been shown to help reduce emotional problems and depression, especially those associated with nervous exhaustion or nervous system problems. Studies have shown that it can be useful in reducing emotional distress, insomnia, uneasiness, and exhaustion. In an attempt to bring the body into balance, it can help people who are nervous and underweight gain weight and those with hormonal irregularities become stabilized.

Depression is a common problem that affects millions of Americans. While some cases of depression involve an imbalance of the neurotransmitters, or chemical messengers, in the brain, other cases involve psychological triggers. Counseling and professional care may be crucial in recovery, but ginseng and other natural remedies may be helpful in mild cases.

- In Europe, ginseng often is prescribed to treat depression, especially in elderly people. Studies conducted in Italy have shown that ginseng helped improve the mood and lift melancholy in older people.

- Other studies have shown that people with more severe emotional problems—those who were hostile, unsociable, and uncooperative—experienced a more positive outlook, and their attention span and level of concentration also improved after taking ginseng.

NOTE: If you are already taking antidepressants, discuss the matter with your doctor before self-prescribing ginseng. Ginseng can reduce the effectiveness of many narcotics and sedatives, probably due to its adaptogenic effects at bringing the body back into balance.

FOR MORE INFORMATION

If you would like to know more about depression, discuss the matter with your health care provider and contact one or more of the following organizations:

Depressives Anonymous
329 East 62nd Street
New York, NY 10021
(212) 689-2600

Depression and Related Affective Disorders Association
Johns Hopkins Hospital
600 North Wolfe Street
Baltimore, MD 21287
(410) 955-4647

Depression Awareness, Recognition, and Treatment (DART)
National Institute of Mental Health
9000 Rockville Place
Bethesda, MD 20892
(800) 421-4211

Foundation for Depression and Manic Depression
24 East 81st Street, Suite 2B
New York, NY 10028
(212) 772-3400

National Mental Health Association
1021 Prince Street
Alexandria, VA 22314
(800) 243-2525
(703) 684-7722

**National Depressive and Manic
Depressive Association**
730 North Franklin Street, Suite 501
Chicago, IL 60610
(800) 826-3632
(312) 642-0049

**National Foundation for Depressive
Illness**
P.O. Box 2257
New York, NY 10116
(212) 268-4260

RHEUMATOID ARTHRITIS

Rheumatoid arthritis is a disease in which the body turns against itself. The immune system attacks the joints and organs because it is unable to recognize healthy tissue. Rheumatoid arthritis affects the entire body, causing chronic inflammation of many joints as well as the skin, muscles, blood vessels, and, in rare cases, organs such as the heart and lungs.

In addition to joint problems, rheumatoid arthritis can cause fever, fatigue, weight loss, anemia, and tingling hands and feet. If the organs become involved, complications can include an enlarged spleen, irregular heartbeat, or pleurisy, an inflammation of the membrane covering the lungs.

Ginseng can be helpful in the treatment of rheumatoid arthritis because it encourages the release of the adrenal hormones, including hydrocortisone, which reduce inflammation and pain. While many prescription drugs have adverse side effects and tend to shrink the adrenal glands, ginseng actually reverses adrenal shrinkage. It also boosts the immune system, which helps in the management of the disease.

Ginseng can be combined with other herbs in the treatment of rheumatoid arthritis. Herbs often used in combination with ginseng include:

- Buplerum (*Bupleurum falcatum*)
- Echinacea (*Echinace species*)
- Licorice (*Glycyrrhiza glabra*)
- Turmeric (*Curcuma longa*)
- Yucca (*Yucca species*)

FOR MORE INFORMATION

If you would like more information on rheumatoid arthritis, discuss the matter with your health care provider and contact one or more of the following organizations:

American College of Rheumatology
60 Executive Park South
Suite 150
Atlanta, GA 30329
(404) 633-3777

The Arthritis Foundation
1314 Spring Street, N.W.
Atlanta, GA 30309
(800) 283-7800
(404) 872-7100

National Arthritis and Musculoskeletal and Skin Diseases Information Clearinghouse
9000 Rockville Pike
P.O. Box AMS
Bethesda, MD 20892-2903
(301) 495-4484

SKIN CARE

Ginseng can be used as a cosmetic cream. When it is added to a facial moisturizer, ginseng helps the skin to remain smooth and wrinkle-free. The herb also can help with acne and skin irritation. Some commercial cosmetics contain ginseng (often in combination with vitamin E and aloe vera).

- Ginseng has been shown to slow baldness associated with excessive production of scalp oil. In a study of one hundred people with scalp inflammation and dandruff, symptoms gradually disappeared over the course of several months in all participants after they applied a lotion containing Siberian ginseng to their scalps and consumed oral Silberian ginseng extract. The oil production returned to normal and their hair stopped falling out.

SURGICAL RECOVERY

Surgery is a significant stress on the body, and a number of studies have demonstrated the benefits of using ginseng during recovery from surgery. In fact some plastic surgeons now recommend that their patients take ginseng for two weeks after surgery to speed healing. Consider the evidence:

- In a study involving 120 postoperative gynecological patients, 60 were given ginseng daily and 60 others received a placebo. Those given the ginseng experienced a significant increase in their levels of hemoglobin, protein, and hematocrit (a percentage of red blood cells in the total blood volume)—all of which are measures of recovery. A similar study done in Korea also found patients recovered more quickly after surgery if they took ginseng.

As you know from reading the previous sections, ginseng can be very effective at treating a number of health problems. The following section, Part 3: Using Ginseng, will help you determine how to customize a ginseng program to meet your specific health needs.

PART THREE

Using Ginseng

CHAPTER 9

How to Buy and Use Ginseng

Ginseng is widely available in drug and health food stores, but finding the right product at the right price can be a bit tricky. Shopping for ginseng can be intimidating to a novice: What type of ginseng do you want: American or Asian? Korean or Japanese? And in what form do you want it: A raw root or dried powder? A tincture or tea?

There are many ways you can purchase ginseng; you can buy whole roots from a Chinese herbalist in the nearest city's Chinatown district, or you can go to the local pharmacy or health food store and pick up a bottle of neatly packaged capsules or tinctures. While the best way to be sure you're getting pure, unadulterated ginseng is to prepare your own products from roots, most people don't feel they have the time or expertise to take on the challenge. Fortunately, you can buy high-quality ginseng products commercially, if you know what to look for.

Before you buy, you need to understand the grades, varieties, and forms of ginseng, and you need to appreciate the problems with adulteration and mislabeling that sometimes occur with its marketing and sale. This chapter will help you become a more savvy consumer of ginseng so that you can get the best product for the best price.

MAKING THE GRADE

Ginseng comes in a variety of grades, depending on the root's age, color, density, taste, and shape.

AGE

Generally, the older the root at the time of harvest, the more expensive it is (and the greater its medicinal value). Most high-quality roots are harvested at six to twelve years of age. A ginseng root needs to be at least four years old. Between the fourth and sixth years, the root doubles in weight, and the amount of ginsenosides the root doubles, usually by the end of the sixth year. After that time, the root will continue to grow and accumulate more ginsenosides, but at a slower pace. Some of the oldest roots have been found to be 100 to 200 years old. As mentioned earlier, the age of the root can be determined by counting the number of ridges or scars on the root's neck; it gets one ridge for every year. (If you buy whole roots, be sure the neck section at the top of the root is present so that you can assess its quality; many inferior roots are sold with their necks removed.)

COLOR

All ginseng is naturally white or pale yellow. Roots are steamed to get the reddish color, they tend to be pricier than white roots because higher-quality roots are usually the ones selected for steaming and because the steaming process is believed to enhance ginseng's medicinal value. (This is not a hard-and-fast rule, since average or inferior-grade roots can be steamed red and remain inferior to a high-quality white root.) The best white ginseng is actually a very pale yellow.

DENSITY

A good white root should be quite hard; a red root should be crystalline, deep in color, and hard and brittle. When analyzed, red ginseng has been found to have the same major ginsenosides as white ginseng, plus four additional ginsenosides: Rg2, Rg3, Rh1 and Rh2.

TASTE

Whether white or red, a good root should have a robust flavor, bitter with a slight sweetness; bland roots are inferior.

SHAPE

Good roots are relatively straight with branches (giving it the human form); curled roots are considered lower quality. The tails or rootlets growing from the branches are considered the least potent forms of ginseng and are the cheapest.

GINSENG'S REPUTATION BY TYPE

While this grading system may seem complex, ginsengs from different countries have earned distinct reputations for quality. Of course, herbs will differ in quality within each type, but these general profiles may help you determine which types of ginseng might be best for you.

CHINESE GINSENG

Chinese ginseng is considered the best type marketed in the West, but it is usually available only from Asian herbalists and suppliers. In China, more than 5,000 tons of ginseng are produced a year. In parts of rural China, almost every community has a ginseng patch in a communal garden. The quality ranges from outstanding to mid-level. There are several types of Chinese roots.

- *Wild Tung Pei Ginseng.* This form grows wild or uncultivated in Chinese forests. It is quite rare; only about four or five pounds of it are found each year. Each gram can cost $500 to $600 or more. This grade of ginseng isn't available for sale in the United States.

- *Yi Sun Ginseng.* This is a semiwild form of ginseng. To prepare yi sun, growers plant high-grade seedlings in natural forests where they grow for eight to twelve years. The root, which is similar to wild ginseng but somewhat less potent, is one of the best forms available in the United States; it can cost hundreds of dollars an ounce, but the prices fluctuate with the market.

- *Shiu Chu Ginseng.* This is a widely available, good-quality root. A cultivated root, it costs about $50 an ounce, or about $3 to $7 per root, depending on size and overall quality. **The roots usually are steamed to create a red color.**

- *Kirin Ginseng.* This cultivated ginseng root is named after Kirin Province, where it is grown. This form of ginseng costs about 75 percent of what Shiu Chu ginseng costs. It is the type commonly used in commercially prepared ginseng products; it is of medium quality.

- *Odds and Ends.* These types of ginseng are the small roots, broken pieces, and tails, which are trimmed off the roots and ground into root powders and extracts and then used in capsules, tablets, teas, and other products not involving whole roots. They contain high levels of ginsenosides and have medicinal value, but they are considered inferior to whole roots.

AMERICAN GINSENG

American ginseng is widely available, although much of it is exported to China and Asia. American ginseng is available in wild, semiwild, and cultivated forms.

- *Wild American Ginseng.* This type is not as rare as wild Asian ginseng, although it is considered an endangered species. Wild American ginseng would not be so rare if the early American settlers had used the Native American method of harvesting herbs. The Native Americans waited to harvest the root until the ginseng plant bore fruit, then they planted the seeds in the hole where the root was removed. This method attempted to maintain the natural order of the forest. Wild American ginseng is not available in stores or through catalogs. Because of the plant's status as an endangered species, ethical companies sell only semiwild ginseng.

- *Semiwild American Roots.* These became popular in the late 1980s, when growers began to transplant seedlings into a natural forest habitat, much like the Chinese yi sun ginseng. Some semiwild growers use pesticides and fungicides on their roots, while others grow organically. Semiwild roots are considered more potent than cultivated roots.

- *Cultivated American Ginseng.* This is the most common form. Ginseng has been grown in the United States for hundreds of years, primarily in Wisconsin and Michigan. The herb grows well in these areas because of the cool, moist summers and freezing winters. About 95 percent of the nearly 800,000 pounds of American ginseng grown each year is exported to China.

- *Red American Ginseng.* This variety is formed the same way as Asian red ginseng, by steaming. Red American ginseng is usually a bit more expensive than white American ginseng. Some people question the practice of steaming American ginseng because it increases the root's warming properties, negating the herb's medicinal value as a cooling agent.

KOREAN GINSENG

Korean ginseng can be quite good, ranging in quality from the equivalent of the Chinese shiu chu down to inferior products.

Some Korean roots are grown in the wild, but these roots rarely appear in the Western herb market.

The best Korean ginseng is red ginseng; it is classified as Heaven Grade, Earth Grade, and Man Grade. The Korean government carefully regulates the Korean ginseng market so most products are of reasonably good quality.

When buying Korean ginseng, look for a tin bearing the seal of the Office of Monopoly in Seoul; some merchants try to pass off poor-quality roots from Hong Kong as authentic Korean red ginseng. Korea also produces midquality white ginseng as well as the broken pieces, tails, and other scraps used to make extracts and other products. As a tonic, Korean ginseng is believed to tone both the yin and the yang, while Chinese ginseng is said to stimulate yang less, making it better for long-term use.

JAPANESE GINSENG

In general terms, Japanese ginseng is of average to poor quality. While some Japanese roots can be of superior quality—as good as the best of the Korean ginseng—these high-quality roots rarely appear in the Western market. Japanese ginseng may be steamed so that it appears red. Most low-quality Japanese roots are shipped to Hong Kong, where they are sold as imitation Korean red ginseng.

SIZING UP A ROOT

Ginseng quality and price depends on the size of the root in addition to the country of origin. Ginseng roots can be sold individually or in packages weighing a unit of measure known as a catty. (A catty equals 600 grams, or slightly more than 1¼ pounds.) The roots are classified into sizes, based on how many roots would equal a given weight. For example, Earth Grade 15 means 15 roots would equal a catty, while Earth Grade 20 means 20 roots to the catty. Within the same grade, the larger the root (the lower the number), the better the herb. In other words, Earth Grade 15 is considered superior to Earth grade 20.

Unfortunately, not every herb seller uses this system. Some herbalists use a grading system with #1, #2, #3, and so on to denote root quality. Under this system, a #1 root is superior in quality to a #2 root. When buying roots, the most important issue is to fully understand the grading system used by the root seller with whom you are dealing.

However, the overall grade—Heaven, Earth, Man—is a better indication of a root's medicinal value. In other words, a small root of Heaven Grade (Heaven Grade 25) would be of better quality than a large root of Earth Grade (Earth Grade 15).

COMPARING COMMERCIAL PRODUCTS

You can either buy a whole root and prepare the herb yourself, or you can shop for commercially prepared ginseng products. While consuming unprocessed roots is undoubtedly the best approach from a medicinal

GO WILD!

The wilder the root, the more potent the medicine. For reasons herbalists do not fully understand, wild or semiwild ginseng roots are more potent than their cultivated kin. In fact, two roots, one semiwild and one cultivated, can have the same ginsenoside content, but the semiwild root has a stronger healing effect on the body.

Often you can identify a cultivated root from a wild one because it may not have the wrinkle or ridge around its crown. Wild roots tend to be harder, denser, and more bitter than the cultivated versions. True wild Chinese ginseng is exceptionally rare and exceptionally expensive at about $240,000 a pound.

point of view, it isn't always practical, especially for someone relatively unfamiliar with working with herbs. Fortunately, commercial ginseng products can offer an easy, inexpensive, and effective way to take ginseng or other herbs. For commercial preparations, always follow the dosage instructions on the product label.

Unfortunately, many commercial products consist of ground root powder made of poor-quality roots. Some companies further diminish the effectiveness of the root by mixing the ginseng powder with a filler, such as lactose. A number of tests on commercial ginseng products have shown that many of them contain few or even no discernible ginsenosides, the active ingredient in ginseng. You may be able to minimize some of this problem by choosing a Chinese or Korean ginseng product that has been imported to the West in its original package. The typical price range for commercial ginseng is about $10 to $12 for a bottle of 30 500-milligram capsules.

Whether you prefer whole roots or commercial products is a matter of personal choice. The following section describes a number of different forms of ginseng; in some cases it also includes information on how to make a product using whole roots.

ARE "STANDARDIZED" PRODUCTS BETTER?

One way to improve your chances of getting a better commercial product is to buy standardized ginseng extract in tablets, capsules or liquid form. Standardization is a way of processing ginseng that guarantees a fixed amount of ginsenosides in every dose.

Of the standardized products on the market, most contain ginsenosides in concentrations of 4 to 7 percent. In France, ginseng products must have at least 2 percent ginsenosides to be officially recognized as authentic; in Germany and Switzerland, the amount is 1.5 percent.

The advantage to a standardized product is that it offers some assurance that a product contains medicinal amounts of ginseng. Some herbalists and other health professionals feel more comfortable recommending standardized products because they can more accurately predict the amount of ginsenosides in the product (or the amount of eleutherosides in Siberian ginseng).

There are two main problems with standardization. For one thing, this approach focuses on a single active ingredient, without regard to the many constituents that make a given herb effective. We do not fully understand the synergy among various ingredients in any herb; we should not assume that a single ingredient is as effective alone as it is when combined with the other compounds that occur naturally in the whole plant.

A second problem is that standardization does not assure that the ingredients in a products are of good quality. A product may contain the appropriate amount of ginseng, but the root itself may not be of high quality. If you are concerned about adulteration, you may prefer to buy a standardized product, but don't assume that standardized products are necessarily superior to other forms of ginseng.

WHOLE ROOTS

A slice of root can be cut from the whole, chewed until soft, and swallowed. Most ginseng roots are four or five inches long at the time of harvest. Cut a slice about the thickness of a nickel. Raw roots can be difficult to cut; they can be easier to slice if steamed for a few minutes. (It's best to cut the whole root after steaming; pour honey over the roots to keep them moist and store them in the refrigerator in a sealed container where they can last for several weeks.) The typical dose is one or two slices a day; the typical slice should weigh about one gram. (When weighing slices, use a gram scale, a postage scale, or high-quality kitchen scale; if your scale measures in ounces, keep in mind that there are about thirty grams in an ounce.)

Whole roots are sold in Chinese stores and through the mail. (See pages 229–233). They are also available presliced. Buying and eating whole roots offers the assurance that you are consuming real, unadulterated ginseng. When buying whole roots, expect that the quality of the plant is reflected in the price. For example, American ginseng can range from about $10 to $60 per ounce, depending on the grade.

POWDERED GINSENG

Many people find it easier to use ginseng after the root has been ground into powdered form. You can grind it yourself using a coffee or seed grinder, then consume one to two grams of powder a day by mixing it with warm water, tea, wine, or another beverage, or by preparing gelatin capsules (available at health food stores). As you might expect, it is easier to digest ginseng in powdered form than as a whole root.

Ginseng powder is commercially available, but you have more information about the quality of the product you are using if you prepare it yourself. Powdered ginseng is sometimes mixed with other herbs to create herbal formulas designed to create a specific healing effect. Chinese formulas or patent formulas based on ancient recipes are sold in Chinese stores and health food stores. Before self-prescribing a patent formula, you should talk to a professional herbalist. While the product should be designed to minimize any negative side effects, you want to be sure you use the right formula for your particular needs.

TINCTURES

Tinctures are concentrated alcohol extracts that are sold in small bottles with dropper tops. The usual dose is a few drops of tincture mixed with tea or another beverage. In most products, the concentration is one part ginseng to five parts alcohol listed as (1:5 on the label). Ginseng enters the body fastest when consumed as a tincture since the various ingredients have already been broken down in the tincture-making process.

TEAS

Commercially prepared instant ginseng teas are usually made from the roots, leaves, or flowers of the plant and have little or no medicinal value. If you want a strong form of ginseng tea, you should consider making it yourself.

Ginseng is too expensive to prepare in the same way as a regular tea. The Chinese prepare ginseng tea in a ginseng cooker, which works like a double boiler. (They are available at Chinese herb stores and by mail; see pages 229–233.) The cookers are designed to prevent the tea from boiling, which can destroy some of the active ingredients. A homemade alternative to the ginseng cooker is to put the ginseng and water in a sealed airtight baggie or jar and place it in a large pot of boiling water. Use six grams of ginseng root or one teaspoon of powdered ginseng in a cup of water, and cook the tea for about two hours. Drink half the tea as a daily dose.

Rather than discard the root after preparing the tea, cut the slices into smaller pieces and repeat the process. The first preparation extracts the active ingredients from the outer root; the second batch draws from the innermost part of the root. You can prepare a third batch using the same roots, for a total of three preparations (or six servings). If you don't like the taste of the tea, you might want to improve the flavor by brewing the ginseng with ginger powder or several slices of ginger root (available at most grocery stores).

GRANULES

To prepare granules, a manufacturer brews a huge vat of tea. The water is then evaporated and the residue is made into dissolvable granules. To prepare tea, all you have to do is add the appropriate amount of granules to hot water. Granules are available from herbalists. Ginseng is not commonly used in granule form.

WINE

Chinese healers sometimes prescribe preparations of ginseng wine. To prepare ginseng wine, thinly slice three ounces of ginseng root and soak it in a wine of your choosing for about six weeks. Store the wine in the refrigerator and shake it every day or two. Consume no more than one ounce a day. (Ginseng wine should be viewed as a medicine, not a typical alcoholic beverage.)

CANDIES, CHEWING GUM, AND OTHER PRODUCTS

A number of other products, from soup flavoring to cigarettes, soda to ice cream, have ginseng added to them to enhance their healing reputation. Don't rely on any of these products to have any tonic or healing effects, although they might serve as a slight pick-me-up.

THE PROBLEM OF ADULTERATION: WHEN GINSENG ISN'T GINSENG

Because of its expense, ginseng is a common target for consumer scams and product adulteration. Throughout history, unscrupulous herb merchants have substituted

CAVEAT EMPTOR

When it comes to buying ginseng, don't hunt for bargains. The classic consumer adage holds true in the world of herbs: If a deal sounds too good to be true, it probably is.

Pass on the specials and two-for-one deals sometimes offered by manufacturers. Bargain-priced herbs almost always indicate inferior herbs. High-quality ginseng is expensive because it takes years to cultivate and grow the plant. A manufacturer can't cut costs without cutting corners. For ginseng to be potent enough to be of medicinal value, chances are good that it won't be sold at rock-bottom prices. Expect to pay at least $10 to $12 for a bottle of 30 500 milligram capsules.

less costly herbs for ginseng in herbal formulas and powdered herbs. Because of the problems with dishonest merchants, ginseng roots often are bought and sold whole so that buyers can determine the quality of the root they are buying.

Today ginseng is often sold as capsules or tinctures, which makes determining the quality and quantity of herb in a product much more difficult. In the late 1970s, several researchers analyzed the contents of more than fifty commercial ginseng products. They found that 25 percent contained no ginseng and another 35 percent contained so little ginseng that they were of no medicinal value.

The problem of mislabeling continues. In November 1995 *Consumer Reports* magazine published an analysis of ten ginseng products. A legitimate ginseng product should contain 3 to 6 percent ginsenosides by weight. Of the products tested, six had less than 3 percent ginsenosides, probably because the products used excessive amounts of fillers and binders. Without the appropriate levels of ginsenosides, a ginseng product cannot provide the promised health benefits.

COMPARING PRODUCT PRICES

It is very difficult to compare prices of ginseng products. Browsing the products on

GROWING GINSENG

Ginseng is exceedingly difficult to find growing in the wild. In fact, ginseng has been called "the root that hides from man" because it naturally grows in the deep forest in rich, moist soils, where it can be exceedingly difficult to identify and harvest.

Unfortunately, ginseng also is a challenge to grow efficiently; it requires painstaking cultivation and is quite vulnerable to attack by pests and disease, especially fungi.

Traditional Asian methods of cultivation call for frequent transplanting of the ginseng to fresh beds and only using beds that have not had ginseng growing in them for twelve years. Because of the high demand for the herb, these ancient practices are no longer used, and recently ginseng crops have been subject to increasing amounts of disease; in fact, as much as one-third of Chinese crop is damaged by disease.

Ginseng can be a finicky plant to grow. The plant needs well-drained, clay-based soil containing high amounts of organic matter, such as leaf mold. Ideally, the plant grows on gently sloping forested land facing the north. The soil should be a slightly acidic, with a pH of 5.5.

> Researchers have found that the roots grow best when the shading allows 20 percent of the light to filter through.
>
> Ginseng is easy to find at the local health food store or pharmacy, but it is extraordinarily difficult to find ginseng in the wild.

the shelf can be baffling: Products are sold in different doses, weights, potencies, and numbers of capsules per bottle. You can pay a little—or a lot—per gram of ginseng, and the actual value of a given product may not be clear unless you perform a couple of quick calculations.

When comparing prices, your goal is to compare the price per gram of two or more products.

- First, you want to determine the amount of actual ginseng in the bottle. To calculate this, multiply the number of milligrams by the number of capsules or tablets in the bottle. For example, a product containing 30 pills, each containing 100 milligrams of ginseng, would contain 3,000 milligrams of ginseng (or 3 grams):

30 pills × 100 mg = 3,000 milligrams
3,000 mg ÷ 1,000 mg per gram = 3 grams

- To determine the cost per gram, divide the cost of the product by the number of grams. For example, if the sample product cost $10 for 30 grams, the cost of the product would be 33¢ per gram:

$10 ÷ 30 grams = 33¢ per gram

If a manufacturer simply grinds up dried root and puts the powder into capsules, you can compare prices by comparing the costs per gram using these calculations. However, many manufacturers use an extraction process to concentrate the active ingredients of ginseng powders, making the product more uniform and more potent.

In most cases, the extraction ratio ranges from 2:1 to 5:1, indicating how many grams of ginseng powder were used to create the extract. The higher the ratio, the greater the concentration of active ingredients in the extracted root. For a product with a 5:1 extraction ratio, the active ingredients found in five grams of ginseng have been concentrated in one gram of ginseng extract.

Some companies do not indicate on the product label what the extraction ratio is, making it impossible to compare potencies. If a manufacturer does list the extraction ratio, take that number into account when performing your calculation. For example, a product containing 100 mg capsules of ginseng prepared from a 5:1 ratio would contain the equivalent of 500 mg ginseng per capsule.

When trying to assess the value of a product made with ginseng extract, you must first determine how much ginseng is in the product, then determine the cost per gram. Ideally, you should look for products that provide full disclosure of product weight and extraction information. The best companies clearly label their products with the total amount of ginseng the product contains and whether it is an extract.

CHAPTER 10 .

Designing Your Ginseng Program

Now you know that ginseng can boost your energy levels, help you combat stress, reinforce your immune system, and improve your overall health. You also know that ginseng is not only effective but also remarkably free of the side effects often associated with traditional medicines used to achieve these health benefits.

If you are ready to join the millions of Americans who are already benefiting from the regular use of ginseng, this chapter will help you devise your own ginseng program. The information here draws on a combination of thousands of years of Chinese tradition and the best of modern science.

Of course, you know that ginseng is not a miracle cure. While ginseng may be an important piece of your treatment plan, you should use the herb as only one part of a comprehensive strategy for your overall health. Before embarking on any self care regimen, you should discuss any health concerns with your doctor or health care professional.

IS GINSENG RIGHT FOR YOU?

Ginseng is a very safe herb with few side effects, even when it is taken in large doses or over a long period of time. Like any other herb, ginseng is not unquestionably safe under every circumstance, but it is much safer than most prescription drugs used to achieve the same physical effects.

In animal studies researchers have found that a harmful dose of ginseng is at least 1,000 times the effective dose, or an amount equal to a person eating three to four pounds of ginseng roots at a single sitting. In another study, a French researcher tried to give laboratory mice enough ginseng to cause adverse side effects; except for their stomachs becoming distended due to overeating, the rats did not experience any negative effects.

One reason ginseng may have so few side effects is that its active ingredients are not toxic. Researchers have determined that the ginsenosides in ginseng are about ten times less toxic than the caffeine in coffee and tea.

Despite its reputation as a safe herb, some people do experience unwanted side effects when taking ginseng. In most cases, side effects do not show up unless a person takes an excessive dose of ginseng (more than nine or ten grams a day). Problems associated with excessive ginseng intake include diarrhea, diminished libido, earaches, headaches, high blood pressure, insomnia, itchy skin, rashes, low white blood counts, nausea, nosebleeds, palpitations, and vomiting. Most side effects don't show up unless high doses are taken for an extended period of time.

Despite the slight chance of negative side effects, ginseng is not an herb that should be used by everyone. Keep the following restrictions in mind when designing your ginseng program:

- If you have high blood pressure, do not use ginseng without discussing the matter with your doctor. The herb can increase blood pressure.

- If you have diabetes, do not use ginseng without carefully monitoring your blood-sugar levels and discussing the use of the herb with the physician or endocrinologist treating the disease. Ginseng can lower blood-sugar levels, which need to be maintained at a steady level to manage diabetes.

- If you are taking medications for the treatment of schizophrenia, depression, bipolar disorder (manic depression), or extreme anxiety, do not use ginseng without talking the matter over with your doctor or psychiatrist. Do not use ginseng if you are taking monoamine oxidase inhibitors (MAOIs). Ginseng can be overly stimulating when used in combination with these drugs.

- If you are taking other prescription drugs, do not use ginseng or any other herb without discussing the matter with your doctor. Herbs and prescription drugs can interact, sometimes with one delaying the absorption of the other. Do not use ginseng if you are taking anticoagulant medications, such as Warfarin.

MAKING GINSENG WORK FOR YOU

After reading this far, you may be convinced that ginseng would help to enhance your life and improve your health. But ginseng is not a tonic for all circumstances; the right type of roots must be taken by the right person in the right way. If the herb is used properly, you can enjoy its healthful benefits; if it is used in the wrong way, it will not be effective, and it may even have negative effects.

If you have decided to try ginseng to maximize your energy and improve your health, you need to learn how to use it most effectively. Keep in mind that research shows that the dosage and usage information are the same for the treatment of most conditions. In other words, the key points listed in this chapter apply whether you're using ginseng to increase your energy or to enhance your immune system.

You may have a number of questions about the practical use of the herb. The following information will help you customize your ginseng program.

How much is enough?

Commercial ginseng products have specific dosage recommendations on the package; always follow the manufacturer's advice and do not exceed the recommended dose. The generic dose recommended by Western herbalists is about one gram daily. This can be in the form of two to three pills, a few cups of tea, one to three drops of tincture or extract, or a nickel-thick slice of raw ginseng root.

If possible, it is best to divide the daily dose, taking half in the morning and half later in the day. Taking more than three grams of ginseng daily can be counterproductive, since it increases the risk of side effects and it is difficult for the body to absorb and use.

To some degree, it's up to you to fine-tune the appropriate dose that best meets your individual needs based on experimenting with different doses and how they make you feel. Always begin with a low level and gradually increase it until you notice the positive effects you seek.

When should I take ginseng?

It is best to take ginseng at least one-half hour before a meal so that the process of digestion does not interfere with the absorption of the active ingredients.

If you are taking one capsule per day, try to take it in the morning with water. If possible, avoid taking ginseng after dinner because it can be so stimulating that it disturbs a good night's rest.

How long should I take ginseng?

For most people, the optimal way of using ginseng is to use it for three or four weeks at a time. (This is sometimes referred to as a course.) You can then discontinue using the herb for one to two weeks, then take another course, if necessary.

Keep in mind, however, that some people can benefit from using ginseng continuously. For example, older people and those recovering from illness or a prolonged period of stress may prefer to take a maintenance dose of about one gram on an ongoing basis. Chinese tradition holds that young and healthy people need only an occasional one-month course of ginseng, the sick, injured, and elderly people can take it on an ongoing basis.

How long will I have to take ginseng before I feel better?

Some people feel the effects of taking ginseng right away, while others may not notice any changes at all. In general, the more tired and run down you are or the more anxious and distraught, the more you will notice a return to your normal state of balance. As you might expect, effects of taking ginseng at higher doses for shorter periods of time will be more noticeable than taking ginseng at lower doses for longer periods.

Should I vary the type of ginseng I use based on the season?

Chinese herbalists often recommend that a person use Asian ginseng during the cold winter months (because Asian ginseng is warming) and American ginseng during the hot summer months (because American ginseng is cooling). This can be one of several factors you consider when comparing the types of ginseng and which product you think is right for you. (For more information on choosing which type of ginseng to take, see page 218.)

How can I use ginseng as a short-term pick-me-up?

If you want to use ginseng as a stimulant to counteract fatigue or to build strength after an illness, take two to three grams a day, divided between morning and evening doses.

How should I store my ginseng?

Ginseng is best stored as whole roots rather than cut or powdered. In whatever form, it should be kept in a dry, airtight container; moisture can cause ginsenosides to break down. Studies have shown that after three years, a sample of white ginseng had 27 percent fewer ginsenosides and a sample of red ginseng had 12 percent

fewer ginsenosides than the samples
had before storage.

**Should I avoid any foods or medications
when taking ginseng?**

Yes. To avoid overstimulation, you
should avoid caffeine and other
stimulants. The combination of ginseng
and other stimulating agents can cause
overexcitement. If you are taking any
medications, check with your doctor
before using ginseng, or any other herb.

**Is ginseng best taken alone or as part of
a formula?**

Ginseng can be used either way. In
Oriental medicine, ginseng often is
combined with other herbs as part of an
overall remedy. In fact, ginseng is
included in more than one out of every
four classical Chinese prescriptions.
When ginseng is added to a treatment
for a specific disease, it is not
considered the curative agent, but it is

included to support the person's overall health and promote balance and healing throughout the body.

Is ginseng helpful in the treatment of ongoing chronic conditions such as rheumatoid arthritis or chronic fatigue syndrome?

No, although ginseng may be included as part of a Chinese formula used to treat a chronic condition. Ginseng actually may mask an illness or nutrient deficiency that is causing a chronic condition. If you have a chronic health problem, consult your doctor or a professional herbalist; do not rely on ginseng alone to correct the problem.

What should I look for on a product label to make sure a commercial product is of good quality?

It can be difficult to determine whether a commercial ginseng preparation is of high quality. Look for a product labeled as *Panax ginseng* or *Panax quinquefolius* standardized to 4 to 7 percent ginsenosides. While this label does not guarantee a product of high quality, it provides a measure of quality control that other products do not. Of course, if you want to be sure you're getting the best ginseng possible, you can order whole roots by mail or from a professional herbalist. (For information on mail-order companies and suppliers, see pages 229–233.)

I have read stories about ginseng causing birth defects. Are the stories true?

No. A number of stories circulated in 1990 about a Canadian baby being born with excessive body hair and hormonal imbalances because the mother drank tea labeled "Siberian ginseng" during her pregnancy. Researchers who followed the study found that the beverage the woman drank contained Chinese silk vine, an herb that is sometimes substituted for genuine

ginseng in commercial products. Furthermore, the researchers found that the herb did not have any bearing on the infant's condition. Before using ginseng or any other herb during pregnancy, discuss the matter with your obstetrician.

WHICH TYPE OF GINSENG IS BEST FOR YOU?

As you know, different types of ginseng affect the body in different ways. The type of ginseng you should use depends on the reason you are taking the herb. The following summary should help you choose which of the three major types of ginseng is best for you.

ASIAN GINSENG: STIMULATING, HOT, AND YANG

Asian ginseng tends to be much more stimulating than either American or Siberian ginseng. Asian ginseng "warms" the body by stimulating the hormonal system. Red ginseng is "hotter," or more potent, than white because the method of preparation slightly alters the chemical composition of the root.

Who Should Use Asian Ginseng. Asian ginseng is a good choice for people who are tired, run down, recovering from illness, or for elderly people whose hormonal systems are not functioning as well as they once did. Some athletes who exercise strenuously use Asian ginseng to help fuel their workouts. In China, it is used to revive dying patients and to treat impotence.

Who Should Avoid Asian Ginseng. Asian ginseng is not a good choice for people who are high-strung, anxious, or nervous. It is not recommended for children, women, or people with Type A personalities. (Asian ginseng, particularly red ginseng, can make some women experience a change in their normal menstrual cycle.) Asian ginseng is not a good choice for people who use other stimulants (such as caffeine and refined sugars) on a regular basis. As a general rule, Asian ginseng is not recommended for healthy people under age forty because it can be too stimulating.

AMERICAN GINSENG: CALMING, COOL AND YING

American ginseng tends to be calming. It helps balance the body and relieve the symptoms of stress. American ginseng contains high levels of certain ginsenosides that tend to depress rather than stimulate the central nervous system.

Who Should Use American Ginseng. American ginseng is a good choice for people who need only a slight increase in energy or help in reducing and managing the physical challenges of stress. It is usually a good choice for women, and should not affect a woman's menstrual cycle.

Who Should Avoid American Ginseng. American ginseng is not the best choice for people who are elderly, run down, or fatigued.

SIBERIAN GINSENG: THE BALANCED APPROACH

Siberian ginseng is considered to be the most adaptogenic of the ginsengs. It is a good all-purpose ginseng, suitable for most people at most times of life.

Who Should Use Siberian Ginseng. Siberian ginseng can be used by almost anyone even for long periods of time without risk of harmful effects. It is especially helpful for people under stress, because stress can present unpredictable symptoms in the body. Siberian ginseng is ideal for people who are generally healthy but would like to use the herb as part of an energizing or rejuvenating program.

Who Should Avoid Siberian Ginseng. Because of the moderating influence, there are no particular people who should not use of this species of ginseng. However, it is milder than both Asian and American ginseng, so a person with extreme symptoms who fits the classic description of a good candidate for one of the other types of ginseng might be better served by another species.

Of course, the choice of which type of ginseng is right for you is a matter of personal preference. Your specific needs may even change from week to week or month to month; you might want to try one type of ginseng for a few weeks or a month on a trial basis. If after that time you feel uncomfortable with the changes you have experienced, you might want to switch to another type of ginseng. For example, if you try Asian ginseng and find it too stimulating, you might want to switch to Siberian ginseng and see if you can maintain the energizing benefits of the herb, without experiencing any symptoms of overstimulation.

The goal, according to the traditional Chinese philosophy of the world, is to achieve a balance between your yin and yang. These complementary forces oppose one another. When one increases, the other decreases and vice versa. For balanced health, you need balanced yin and yang, and ginseng can help you achieve this goal.

In the following section of the book you

will find resources that can help you put your ginseng program into action. It includes lists of organization of interest, mail-order sources of herbs, web sites of interest, as well as a comprehensive bibliography.

ARE YOU YIN OR YANG?

Traditional Chinese medicine is a system of healing that relies on thousands of years of medical experience. It is based on the teachings set forth in *Nei Ching, The Yellow Emperor's Classic of Internal Medicine.* The book contains the dialogue between a legendary Chinese furniture maker and his court physician. It is based on the concept of balance, so that the *qi* or life energy can flow freely throughout the body. In traditional Chinese medicine there are certain common signs of deficiency in yin or yang:

SIGNS OF YANG DEFICIENCY

- Aversion to cold

- Chilly hands and feet

- Plentiful urine

- Clear urine

- Loose stools

- Dark tongue

- Slow pulse

SIGNS OF YIN DEFICIENCY

- Flushed face
- Hot hands and feet

- Dry mouth and throat

- Night sweats

- Premature ejaculation in men

- Dry, red tongue

- Fast pulse

Organizations of Interest

American Association of Naturopathic Physicians
601 Valley Street
Suite 105
Seattle, WA 98109
(206) 298-0125
www.naturopathic.org

This organization can provide referrals to naturopathic physicians who are members of the association. In addition, the group offers brochures and background information on naturopathic medicine.

American Botanical Council
P.O. Box 144345
Austin, TX 78714-4345
(512) 331-8868
(800) 373-7105
www.herbalgram.org

The council is a nonprofit educational organization dedicated to providing information on herbs to practitioners of herbal medicine and the public. It also publishes the quarterly journal, *HerbalGram*, an herb magazine with a readable but strongly scientific focus. Cost: $25 per year.

American Herb Association
P.O. Box 1673
Nevada City, CA 95959
(530) 265-9552

The association provides its members with a quarterly newsletter that includes updates on current studies, reviews of books and videos, and legal news and controversies regarding herbs. It also offers directories of mail-order herb products.

Ginseng Research Board of Wisconsin
16-H Menard Plaza
Wausau, WI 54401
(715) 845-7300

The board promotes the use of Wisconsin ginseng and offers a brochure outlining the benefits of using ginseng. The board also provides a seal of quality to ginseng growers who meet the required standard; as part of the qualification process, the board tests items off the shelf.

Herb Research Foundation
1007 Pearl Street, Suite 200
Boulder, CO 80302
(303) 449-2265
www.herbs.org

The foundation has a medicinal library that provides packets of information about individual herbs, including ginseng. Standard information packets cost $7 for nonmembers, or $5 for members. The foundation does not sell herbs.

Institute for Traditional Medicine
2017 Southeast Hawthorne
Portland, OR 97214
(503) 233-4907
www.europa.com/~itm

The nonprofit institute provides educational materials and conducts research on natural healing for health professionals and interested consumers.

Mail-Order Sources of Herbs

Blessed Herbs
109 Barrie Plains Road
Oakham, MA 01068
(800) 489-4372

Dabney Herbs
P.O. Box 22061
Lewisville, KY 40252
(502) 893-5198
www.dabneyherbs.com

Earth's Harvest
14385 S.E. Lusted Road
Sandy, OR 97055
(800) 428-3308

East Earth Trade Winds
P.O. Box 493151
Redding, CA 96049-3151
(800) 258-6878
(916) 241-6878 in California
(800) 258-1384
www.snowcrest.net/eetw/

Eclectic Institute
14385 Lusted Road
Sandy, OR 97055
(800) 332-HERB
www.eclecticherb.com

Gardens of the Blue Ridge
P.O. Box 10
Pineola, NC 28662
(704) 733-2417

Great China Herb Company
857 Washington Street
San Francisco, CA 94108
(415) 982-2195

Herbs Etc.
1345 Cerrillos Road
Santa Fe, NM 87505
(800) 634-3727

Herbs of Grace
Division of School of Natural Medicine
P.O. Box 7369
Boulder, CO 80306-7369
(303) 455-8048
www.purehealth.com

Herb-Pharm
P.O. Box 116
William, OR 97544
(503) 846-6262

Institute for Traditional Medicine
2017 SE Hawthorne
Portland, OR 97214
(800) 544-7504
www.europa.com/~itm

Mayway U.S.A.
1338 Mandela Parkway
Oakland, CA 94607
(510) 208-3113
www.mayway.com

McZand Herbal Inc.
P.O. Box 5312
Santa Monica, CA 90409
(310) 822-0500
(800) 800-0405
www.zand.com

Meridian Traditional Herbal Products
44 Linden Street
Brookline, MA 02146
(800) 356-6003
(617) 739-2636 in Massachusetts

Nature's Way Products, Inc.
10 Mountain Springs Parkway
Springville, UT 84663
(801) 489-1520
www.naturesway.com

Rainbow Light
207 McPherson Street
Santa Cruz, CA 95060
(800) 635-1233
(800) 227-0555

Turtle Island Herbs
1705 14th Street, # 171
Boulder, CO 80302
(303) 442-2215

White Crane
426 First Street
Jersey City, NJ 07302
(800) 994-3721

Windriver Herbs
P.O. Box 3876
Jackson, WY 83001
(800) 903-HERB

Wise Woman Herbals
P.O. Box 279
Creswell, OR 97426
(800) 532-5219

Web Sites of Interest

The list of organizations of interest on pp. 229–233 contains other web sites of interest.

Algy's Herb Page
www.algy.com/herb/index.html

The Alternative Medicine Homepage
www.pitt.edu/~cbw/altm.html

HealthGate
www.healthgate.com

Institute for Traditional Medicine
www.europa.com/~itm

MedWeb
www.medweb.emory.edu

Winifred Conkling

Yahoo!'s Alternative Medicine Page
**www.yahoo.com/health/
alternative_medicine**

Yahoo! Health: Women's Health
www.yahoo.com/health/women_s_health

Bibliography

BOOKS

Bergner, Paul. *The Healing Power of Ginseng and The Tonic Herbs: The Enlightened Person's Guide*. Rocklin, Calif.: Prima Publishing, 1996.

Dharmananda, S. *The Ginseng Story*. Portland, Ore.: Institute for Traditional Medicine, 1994.

Foster, S. *Asian Ginseng: Panax ginseng*. Austin, Tex.: American Botanical Council, 1991.

Foster, S. *American Ginseng: Panax quinquefolium*. Austin, Tex.: American botanical Council, 1991.

Fulder, Stephen. *The Ginseng Book: Nature's Ancient Healer*. Garden City, NY: Avery Publishing Group, 1996.

Hobbs, Christopher. *Ginseng: The Energy Herb*.

Loveland, Colo.: Botanica Press, 1996.

Kaptchuk, Ted. *The Web That Has No Weaver: Understanding Chinese Medicine.* New York: St. Martin's Press, 1984.

Keville, Kathi. *Ginseng: Everything You Need to Know About This Versatile Herbal Antidote to Stress and Fatigue.* New Canaan, Conn.: Keats Publishing, 1996.

Korngold, Harriet. *Between Heaven and Earth: A Guide to Chinese Medicine.* New York: Ballantine Books, 1991.

Lee, F. C. *Facts About Ginseng: The Elixir of Life.* Elizabeth, N.J.: Hollym International Corp., 1992.

MoraMarco, Jacques. *The Complete Ginseng Handbook: A Practical Guide for Energy, Health, and Longevity.* Chicago, Ill.: Contemporary Publishing Co., 1997.

Murray, Michael T. *Stress, Anxiety, and Insomnia.* Rocklin, Calif.: Prima Publishing, 1995.

Ody, Penelope. *The Herb Society's Complete Medicinal Herbal.* London: Dorling Kindersley, 1993.

Persons, Scott W. *American Ginseng: Green Gold.* Asheville, N.C.: Bright Mountain Books, 1986.

Pritts, Kim Derek. *Ginseng: How to Find, Grow, and Use America's Forest Gold.* Mechanicsburg, Pa.: Stackpole Books, 1995.

Tyler, Varro E. *The Honest Herbal,* 3rd ed. New York: Haworth Press, 1993.

ARTICLES

Baldwin, C. A., Anderson, L. A., and Phillipson, J. D. "What Pharmacists Should Know About Ginseng." *Pharmaceutical Journal* 237, (1986): 583–586.

Buchwald, D., et al. "Chronic Fatigue and the Chronic Fatigue Syndrome: Prevalence in a Pacific Northwest Healthcare System." *Annals of Internal Medicine* 123 (1995): 81–88.

Caso, D. Marasco, F. et al. "Double-blind Study of a Multivitamin Complex Supplemented with Ginseng Extract." *Drugs Exp Clin Res* 22 (1996): 323–329.

Choi, H. K, et al. "Clinical Efficacy of Korean Red Ginseng for Erectile Dysfunction." *International Journal of Impotence Research* 7 (September 1995): 181–186.

Ding, D. Z., et al. "Effects of Red Ginseng on the Congestive Heart Failure and Its Mechanism." *Chung Kuo Chung Hsi I Chieh Ho Tsa Chih* 15 (June 1995): 325–327.

Fulder, S. "Ginseng and the Hypothalamic-Pituitary Control of Stress." *American Journal of Chinese Medicine* 9 (1981): 112–118.

Gillis, C. N. "Panax Ginseng Pharmacology: A Nitric Oxide Link?" *Biochemical Pharmacology* 54 (July 1997): 1–8.

Koren, G. et al. "Maternal Ginseng Use Associated with Neonatal Androgenization." *Journal of the American Medical Association* 264 (1990): 2868.

Liu, M. "Studies on the Anti-Aging and Nootropic Effects of Ginsenoside Rg1 and Its Mechanisms of Actions." *Sheng Li Ko Hsueh Chin Chang* 27 (April 1996): 139–142.

Petkov, V. D., et al. "Effects of Standardized Ginseng Extract on Learning, Memory and

Physical Capabilities." *American Journal of Chinese Medicine* 15 (1987): 19–27.

Phillipson, J. D., and Anderson, L. A. "Ginseng—Quality, Safety and Efficacy?" *Pharmaceutical Journal* 232 (1984): 161–165.

Salvati, G., et al. "Effects of Panax Ginseng C. A. Meyer Saponins on Male fertility." *Panminerva Med* 38 (December 1996): 249–254.

Scaglione, F., et al. "Efficacy and Safety of the Standardized Ginseng Extract G115 for Potentiating Vaccination Against the Influenza Syndrome and Protection Against the Common Cold." *Drugs Exp Clin Res* 22, (1996): 65–72.

See, D. M., et al. "In Vitro Effects of Echinacea and Ginseng on Natural Killer and Antibody-Dependent Cell Cytotoxicity in Healthy Subjects and Chronic Fatigue Syndrome or Acquired Immunodeficiency Syndrome Patients." *Immunopharmacology* 35 (January 1997): 229–235.

Sotaniemi, E. A. "Ginseng Therapy in Non–Insulin-Dependent Diabetic Patients." *Diabetes Care* 18 (October 1995): 1373–1375.

Takahashi, M., and Tokuyama S. "Pharmacological and Physiological Effects of Ginseng on Actions Induced by Opioids and Psychostimulants." *Methods Find Exp Clin Pharmacol* 20 (January–February 1998): 77–84.

Tyler, Varro E. "Ginseng: King of Zing?" *Prevention* 49, (August 1997): 69–72.

Wang, L. C., and Lee, T. F. "Effect of Ginseng Saponins on Exercise Performance in Non-Trained Rats." *Planta Med*, 64 (March 1998): 130–135.

Xiaoguang, C., et al. "Cancer Chemopreventive and Therapeutic Activities of Red Ginseng." *Journal of Ethnopharmacology* 60, (February 1998): 71–78.

Yun, T. K., and Choi, S. Y. "Preventive Effect of Ginseng Intake Against Various Human Cancers: A Case-Control Study on 1987 Pairs." *Cancer Epidemiol Biomarkers Prev* 4 (June 1995): 401–408.

About the Author

Winifred Conkling is a freelance writer specializing in health and consumer topics. She is the author of more than fifteen books on natural medicine and health, including *Secrets of 5-HTP*, *Natural Healing for Children*, *Natural Remedies for Arthritis*, and the forthcoming *Secrets of Ginkgo* and *Secrets of Echinacea*. Her work has been published in a number of national magazines, including *American Health*, *Consumer Reports*, *McCall's*, and *Reader's Digest*. She lives in northern Virginia with her husband and two children.

TAKE YOUR HEALTH INTO YOUR OWN HANDS

ORDER TODAY:

THE ARTHRITIS CURE
Jason Theodosakis, M.D., M.S., M.P.H., Brenda Adderly, M.H.A., and Barry Fox, Ph.D.
___96453-6 $6.50 U.S./$8.50 Can.

SECRETS OF SEROTONIN
Carol Hart
___96087-5 $5.99 U.S./$7.99 Can.

FOODS TO HEAL BY
Barry Fox, Ph.D.
___95987-7 $6.99 U.S./$8.99 Can.

NATURAL HEALING FOR CHILDREN
Winifred Conkling
___96044-1 $6.99 U.S./$8.99 Can.

TAKE THIS BOOK TO THE HOSPITAL WITH YOU
Charles B. Inlander and Ed Weiner
___96326-2 $5.99 U.S./$7.99 Can.

HEADACHES: 47 WAYS TO STOP THE PAIN
Charles B. Inlander and Porter Shimer
___96263-0 $4.99 U.S./$6.50 Can.